# The Flatfoot: Pearls and Pitfalls

*Editor*

J. KENT ELLINGTON

# FOOT AND ANKLE CLINICS

www.foot.theclinics.com

*Consulting Editor*
MARK S. MYERSON

September 2017 • Volume 22 • Number 3

**ELSEVIER**

1600 John F. Kennedy Boulevard • Suite 1800 • Philadelphia, Pennsylvania, 19103-2899

http://www.theclinics.com

**FOOT AND ANKLE CLINICS Volume 22, Number 3**
**September 2017 ISSN 1083-7515, ISBN-13: 978-0-323-54552-5**

Editor: Lauren Boyle
Developmental Editor: Meredith Madeira

*Foot and Ankle Clinics* (ISSN 1083-7515) is published quarterly by Elsevier, Inc., 360 Park Avenue South, New York, NY 10010-1710. Months of issue are March, June, September, and December. Periodicals postage paid at New York, NY, and additional mailing offices. Subscription price per year is $320.00 (US individuals), $489.00 (US institutions), $100.00 (US students), $360.00 (Canadian individuals), $588.00 (Canadian institutions), $215.00 (Canadian students), $460.00 (international individuals), $588.00 (international institutions), and $215.00 (international students). To receive student/resident rate, orders must be accompanied by name of affiliated institution, date of term, and the *signature* of program/residency coordinator on institution letterhead. Orders will be billed at individual rate until proof of status is received. Foreign air speed delivery is included in all *Clinics* subscription prices. All prices are subject to change without notice. **POSTMASTER:** Send address changes to *Foot and Ankle Clinics*, Elsevier Health Sciences Division, Subscription Customer Service, 3251 Riverport Lane, Maryland Heights, MO 63043. **Customer Service: 1-800-654-2452 (US and Canada). From outside of the United States and Canada, call 314-447-8871. Fax: 314-447-8029. E-mail: JournalsCustomerService-usa@ elsevier.com (for print support); JournalsOnlineSupport-usa@elsevier.com (for online support).**

*Reprints.* For copies of 100 or more, of articles in this publication, please contact the Commercial Reprints Department, Elsevier Inc., 360 Park Avenue South, New York, NY 10010-1710. Tel.: 212-633-3874; Fax: 212-633-3820; E-mail: reprints@elsevier.com.

# Contributors

## CONSULTING EDITOR

**MARK S. MYERSON, MD**
Medical Director, The Foot and Ankle Association, Inc, Baltimore, Maryland, USA

## EDITOR

**J. KENT ELLINGTON, MD, MS**
OrthoCarolina Foot & Ankle Institute, Associate Professor, Department of Orthopaedic
Surgery, Carolinas Medical Center, Adjunct Assistant Professor of Biology, UNC
Charlotte, Charlotte, North Carolina, USA

## AUTHORS

**MAURICIO BARBOSA, MD**
Foot and Ankle Orthopedic Fellowship, Northwestern Memorial Hospital, Northwestern
University Feinberg School of Medicine, Chicago, Illinois, USA

**BRUCE COHEN, MD**
OrthoCarolina Foot & Ankle Institute, Charlotte, North Carolina, USA

**WILLIAM HODGES DAVIS, MD**
Medical Director, OrthoCarolina Foot & Ankle Institute, Charlotte, North Carolina, USA

**THEODORA C. DWORAK, MD**
Walter Reed National Military Medical Center, Bethesda, Maryland, USA

**RYAN P. FARMER, MD**
Department of Orthopaedic Surgery, University of Colorado School of Medicine, Aurora,
Colorado, USA

**SAMUEL E. FORD, MD**
Resident Physician, Department of Orthopaedic Surgery, Levine Children's Hospital,
Carolinas HealthCare System, Charlotte, North Carolina, USA

**STEPHEN GREENFIELD, MD**
OrthoCarolina Foot & Ankle Institute, Charlotte, North Carolina, USA

**KENNETH J. HUNT, MD**
Associate Professor and Chief, Foot and Ankle Surgery, Department of Orthopaedic
Surgery, University of Colorado School of Medicine, Aurora, Colorado, USA

**TODD A. IRWIN, MD**
OrthoCarolina Foot & Ankle Institute, Charlotte, North Carolina, USA

**MARCELO E. JARA, MD**
Orthopaedic Department, Clínica Dávila, Santiago, Chile

**ANISH R. KADAKIA, MD**
Associate Professor of Orthopedic Surgery, Director, Foot and Ankle Orthopedic Fellowship, Northwestern Memorial Hospital, Northwestern University Feinberg School of Medicine, Chicago, Illinois, USA

**ARMEN S. KELIKIAN, MD**
Professor of Orthopedic Surgery, Foot and Ankle Orthopedic Fellowship, Northwestern Memorial Hospital, Northwestern University Feinberg School of Medicine, Chicago, Illinois, USA

**JOSHUA A. METZL, MD**
Assistant Professor of Orthopaedics, UC Health Steadman Hawkins Clinic Denver, University of Colorado, Greenwood Village, Colorado, USA

**MARK S. MYERSON, MD**
Medical Director, The Foot and Ankle Association, Inc, Baltimore, Maryland, USA

**EZEKIEL OBURU, MBChB, FRCSEd (Tr and Orth)**
Department of Orthopaedics, University of Nairobi, Nairobi, Kenya

**MILAP S. PATEL, DO**
Foot and Ankle Orthopedic Fellowship, Northwestern Memorial Hospital, Northwestern University Feinberg School of Medicine, Chicago, Illinois, USA

**BRIAN P. SCANNELL, MD**
Associate Professor, Department of Orthopaedic Surgery, Levine Children's Hospital, Carolinas HealthCare System, Charlotte, North Carolina, USA

**JEFFREY D. SEYBOLD, MD**
Twin Cities Orthopedics, Edina, Minnesota, USA

**SCOTT B. SHAWEN, MD**
OrthoCarolina Foot & Ankle Institute, Charlotte, North Carolina, USA

**BRIAN STEGINSKY, DO**
Orthopedic Fellow, Illinois Bone and Joint Institute, Libertyville, Illinois, USA

**ANAND VORA, MD**
Fellowship Director, Orthopaedic Foot and Ankle Surgery, Illinois Bone and Joint Institute, Libertyville, Illinois, USA

# Editorial Advisory Board

# Contents

correction of the hindfoot deformity may result in creating a rigid hindfoot, compromising clinical outcomes. Careful analysis of the lateral radiograph to determine whether the deformity is secondary to the medial column or true peritalar subluxation may allow superior outcomes. Iatrogenic creation of an excessively rigid medial column may lead to significant instability of the remaining joints in the short term and arthrosis in the long term. Medial column arthrodesis should be used selectively to correct gross instability.

Adult acquired flatfoot deformity is a debilitating condition typically affecting middle-aged patients. The multiple components include hindfoot valgus, first ray elevation, medial soft tissue compromise, and forefoot abduction. As the foot becomes unbalanced, the deformity progresses with repetitive loading and time. Untreated patients often need significant reconstructions or extensive arthrodesis after arthritis and joint contractures present. Medializing calcaneal osteotomy is the workhorse operation for correction of hindfoot valgus, reliably correcting deformity with a relatively low complication risk. This article reviews indications, techniques, complications, and outcomes for the medializing calcaneal osteotomy.

In 1975, Evans published an article describing the surgical management of the "calcaneo-valgus deformity," pointing out that the deformity was due to relative shortening of the lateral column of the foot. Correction involved "equalizing" both columns by performing an osteotomy in the neck of the calcaneus 1.5 cm from the calcaneocuboid joint, where a trapezoidal wedge of tricortical bone was placed. Although it was considered a success, there were complications, including sural nerve injury, surgical wound dehiscence, undercorrection, and graft subsidence. The osteotomy grew in popularity. Indications extended to other forms of flatfoot with a low incidence of complications.

Understanding of the complexities of the adult acquired pathologic flatfoot has undergone serious evolution in the past 30 years to an understanding of the subtleties of what causes the different presentations and drives successful treatment. As the treatment of ankle arthritis evolves from fusion to ankle replacement, the need for answers for the difficult patient with valgus degenerative ankle disease begs a look at what causes this form of flatfoot. This article poses the question, is there a subset of patients with "flatfoot" that has little to do with the foot and is all about the ankle?

The overcorrected flatfoot reconstruction is a less common but often difficult sequelae of surgical treatment of the adult acquired flatfoot deformity.

Understanding the patient's symptoms and how they correlate to the procedures performed during the index surgery are paramount to determining the appropriate course of treatment. Patients' symptoms may resemble those seen in the cavovarus foot condition, often secondary to overlengthening of the lateral column or excessive displacement of the calcaneal tuberosity. Osteotomies of the calcaneus, midfoot, and often the first metatarsal may be sufficient to revise the overcorrection. However, hindfoot and/or midfoot arthrodesis may be required in more severe or rigid cases.

In symptomatic patients, undercorrection of a flatfoot deformity can lead to the need for revision surgery to restore functional mechanics and prevent progression of deformity. The underlying cause of undercorrection is failure to fully recognize or understand the extent of the deformity. This article discusses the typical deformities in adult flatfoot and indications for surgical intervention. Also presented are the surgical procedures for the correction of the typical deformity patterns with available outcome statistics and a stepwise algorithm for patient evaluation to assist in treatment and mitigate the risk of undercorrection of deformity.

Malunion remains a common complication after triple arthrodesis, with rates as high as 6% in the reported literature. Careful patient evaluation is critical to determine the location and degree of bony deformity. A stepwise systematic approach to correct hindfoot and midfoot deformity is presented in this article. Few studies have been published to guide foot and ankle surgeons with this difficult clinical scenario, but reports have demonstrated high success rates and low rates of complications after revision triple arthrodesis.

Stage II posterior tibial tendon dysfunction encompasses a wide range of patients with varying degrees of deformity and function. The spectrum of patients can be difficult to treat with a single surgical approach, as evidenced by the wide range of techniques present in the literature. Severity of the deformity, patient functional level, age, and comorbidities must be considered to determine the best course of treatment. This article examines when fusion versus reconstruction is the appropriate treatment of patients with severe stage II posterior tibial tendon dysfunction and its subclassifications.

Pediatric flatfeet are common, are usually asymptomatic, and typically improve over time as young children age. It is critical to differentiate flexible from rigid flatfeet and to assess for associated Achilles contracture with a careful history, physical examination, and initial radiographs. Although there are limited data, nonsurgical management of symptomatic flatfeet, both flexible and rigid, should be exhausted before considering surgical intervention. If patients fail conservative treatment, surgical management with joint-preserving, deformity-corrective techniques is typically used for pediatric flexible flatfeet in conjunction with deformity-specific soft tissue procedures.

# FOOT AND ANKLE CLINICS

**THE CLINICS ARE NOW AVAILABLE ONLINE!**
Access your subscription at:
www.theclinics.com

# Preface

# The Flatfoot: Even After Decades of Work, We Still Need Help Understanding It

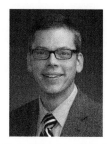

J. Kent Ellington, MD, MS
*Editor*

The flatfoot condition is a very common problem, seen daily in the foot and ankle surgeon's office. Many patients can be treated nonoperatively. If conservative treatment fails, many surgical options exist. Choosing the correct procedure for the correct patient is not as easy as a textbook algorithm may suggest. The identical deformity in one patient may be treated in an entirely different way in another patient. Following flatfoot correction, patients may still have ongoing issues.

This issue dives into details and controversies primarily regarding ideas on how to fix a flatfoot, but also expands our knowledge with what to do if a postoperative flatfoot isn't doing well. I hope these articles by our esteemed authors help you to correct a flatfoot more reliably and teach you how to handle the difficult situation of the unsatisfied patient following an attempted correction.

J. Kent Ellington, MD, MS
OrthoCarolina
Foot & Ankle Institute
2001 Vail Avenue, Suite 200B
Charlotte, NC 28207, USA

*E-mail address:*
kentellingtonfx@gmail.com

Foot Ankle Clin N Am 22 (2017) xiii
http://dx.doi.org/10.1016/j.fcl.2017.06.001
1083-7515/17/© 2017 Published by Elsevier Inc.

# Deltoid Ligament Repair in Flatfoot Deformity

 CrossMark

Ezekiel Oburu, MBChB, FRCSEd (Tr and Orth)[a],*, Mark S. Myerson, MD[b]

## KEYWORDS

- Deltoid ligament reconstruction • Flat foot deformity • Ankle joint mobility

## KEY POINTS

- Deltoid ligament reconstruction allows for joint preservation of the ankle in the setting of a patient with a triple arthrodesis due to a flat foot deformity.
- Although the increased forces that may occur in the ankle joint after a triple arthrodesis cannot be eliminated, reconstruction of the ligament will delay, and may prevent, the onset of arthritis.
- Ligament reconstruction will allow the patient to maintain mobility of the ankle joint.

## INTRODUCTION

In both the acute and the chronic setting the deltoid ligament is not injured frequently as the lateral ligamentous structures. In the flat foot deformity, the medial structures are strained and elongated, and the nature of the injury to the deltoid ligament is chronic, leading to the designation of a stage IV flat foot deformity that was first described by Myerson[1] (**Figs. 1** and **2**). By far, most cases that the authors treat are those in which the posterior tibial tendon (PTT) is ruptured, the foot flat, the deltoid ligament torn, and the ankle joint in varying degrees of valgus. However, it is not that uncommon to find a valgus ankle deformity associated with a normal PTT, but it may be caused by or secondary to the flat foot.

The reducibility and flexibility of the ankle joint determines whether the patient has stage IVA, in which the valgus instability of the joint is reducible, and can benefit from a medial reconstructive procedure. The more common presentation is a patient with stage IVB in which the deformity is fixed and the patient will benefit from an ankle, tibiotalocalcaneal (TTC), or pantalar arthrodesis. Some patients who may not be candidates for surgery may benefit from nonoperative treatment with an Arizona brace.[2]

The authors have nothing to disclose.
[a] Department of Orthopaedics, University of Nairobi, PO Box 2206, Nairobi, Kenya; [b] Institute of Foot and Ankle Reconstruction, 301 St. Paul Place, Baltimore, MD 21202, USA
* Corresponding author.
E-mail address: oburue@gmail.com

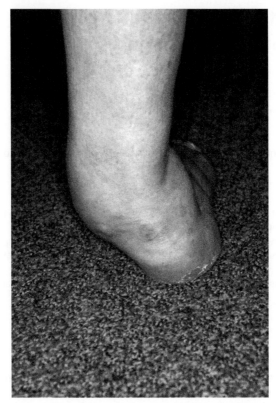

**Fig. 1.** Stage IV posterior tibial tendon dysfunction (PTTD), clinical appearance.

On occasion, the deltoid ligament injury may present in a patient with triple arthrodesis following a flat foot reconstruction. These patients may also benefit from either ligament reconstruction or arthrodesis, depending on the flexibility of the ankle joint. These patients must be approached completely differently because the ankle is in valgus and the hindfoot, including the subtalar joint, is fused, therefore placing the hindfoot in valgus, but the forefoot remains relatively plantigrade. Regardless of the method of ankle correction, as the ankle is brought into neutral, the forefoot will supinate and this must be corrected by plantar flexion of the medical column.

**ANATOMY**

What is it about the deltoid ligament that causes it to rupture in some patients, and for the spring ligament to rupture in others, both occurring with a rupture of the PTT? Why does deltoid rupture not occur more frequently? Certainly, clinicians are accustomed to treating lateral ankle instability, but the anatomy of the deltoid ligament is such that it resists tears and, hence, medial instability. See later discussion of precise anatomy, but here a clinically simple finding is highlighted: the fibers of the deltoid are incredibly thick and strong, blending with the talonavicular capsule distally, making it difficult to tear but also difficult to repair.

The ligament has 2 components: superficial and deep.[3–6] The superficial layer crosses both the ankle and the subtalar joint, whereas the deep layer crosses only

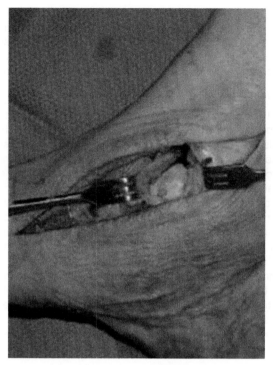

**Fig. 2.** Intraoperative torn deltoid ligament in a patient's PTTD.

the ankle joint. Although this division is specifically used for description purposes to aid in understanding the anatomy, the whole of the ligament is a complex contiguous structure[3] and this differentiation is often not absolutely clear. The deep portion of the ligament is intra-articular but extrasynovial. The individual deep and superficial portions of the ligament have been described as having different components. More recently, Campbell and colleagues[7] described the superficial layer as tibionavicular, tibiospring, tibiocalcaneal, and superficial posterior tibiotalar; and the deep components as deep anterior tibiotalar and deep posterior tibiotalar. This is similar to what has been described by other investigators.[6]

In addition to the medial malleolus, the ligament provides stability against rotatory and valgus forces to the ankle.[8,9] In a cadaveric study, sectioning of the tibiocalcaneal fibers resulted in decreased contact area of up to 43% and increase on contact pressures of up to 30%.[10]

Specifically, patients with stage IV PTT rupture have a hindfoot that is in valgus. The mechanical axis of the leg is shifted medially and, therefore, the ligament eventually becomes incompetent and lengthens.[11,12]

Most patients with stage IV adult acquired flatfoot deformity (AAFD) have a stage B that is associated with varying degrees of ankle arthritis.[2] As previously noted, these patients may not benefit from reconstruction of the ligament and will thus require an arthrodesis, total ankle replacement, or bracing. However, the patient with flexible deformity and the absence of arthritis will benefit from a deltoid ligament reconstruction to prevent valgus loading of the ankle with subsequent development of osteoarthritis. This reconstruction will also help prevent or delay the onset of ankle arthritis after reconstruction of a flat foot deformity, which in this stage is usually a triple arthrodesis. To a great extent, the same principle applies to patients with stage IVB because many of them have early arthritis associated with narrowing of the lateral ankle joint and may benefit from something as simple as a medical translational calcaneus osteotomy or a tibial osteotomy to change the dynamic forces across the joint. These would be combined with a reconstruction of the deltoid ligament.

### Clinical Presentation

In addition to the typical complaints that may be related to PTT rupture, these patients commonly present with ankle pain and a more significant change in the position of the foot. They may also have symptoms of giving way medially when walking on flat surfaces but more so on uneven ground. So, there is little to really distinguish the symptoms of the flat foot associated with a rupture of the PTT from that of a PTT rupture associated with additional pathologic condition of the deltoid.

Clinically, the patient will often but not always have a hindfoot valgus. These patients tend to develop a gastrocnemius contracture that may be masked by the fixed hindfoot deformity and will only become apparent when the hindfoot and the ankle are aligned. Forefoot supination may also be evident when the hindfoot and ankle joint are in alignment.[13]

Clinically, patients with chronic injuries to the deltoid invariably present with pain in the medial gutter that is elicited by palpation of the anterior border of the medial malleolus.[14,15] An anterior drawer sign is negative in these patients. More importantly, the purpose of clinical examination is to establish whether the valgus deformity in the ankle is fixed or flexible, and if there is already established arthritis present in the lateral ankle.

### Imaging

A plain, 3-view, weightbearing radiograph of the ankle may illustrate a valgus tilt of the ankle joint on the AP view (**Figs. 3** and **4**).

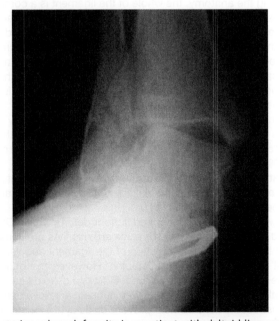

**Fig. 3.** Anteroposterior valgus deformity in a patient with deltoid ligament instability.

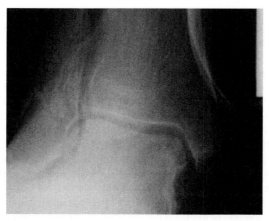

**Fig. 4.** Stress view of the same patient showing reduction of the ankle with varus stress.

Although an MRI may not always be used to help make the diagnosis and may show a tear of the deltoid ligament, the authors have found that examination under fluoroscopy provides dynamic evidence about whether the deltoid ligament is still competent[16] and is particularly helpful to determine flexibility of the ankle.

The importance of this planning cannot be overstated. In many cases, treatment is planned based on clinical findings in which there is marked pain, not along the course of the PTT, but at the medial ankle. Then, under fluoroscopy, the ankle is stable. This does not mean that the deltoid is intact, it means that the ankle is not unstable. The authors are more interested in the ankles that are in valgus on a weightbearing radiograph or those that tilt into valgus on stress testing.

## SURGICAL MANAGEMENT

Some patients may not be candidates for surgery either due to comorbidities or surgery may have to be delayed for uncontrolled reasons; these patients would benefit from the use of Arizona brace. Unlike acute deltoid injuries that may occur in fractures or acute sprains and require either nonoperative care[17–19] or a suture anchor,[20] chronic deltoid ligament injuries require a more elaborate reconstruction.

There are several reconstructive techniques available for deltoid reconstruction. Some are more relevant in the acute setting[20–22] and others are more appropriate in the chronic setting.[23–25] It is important recognize that the standard reconstructive procedures that are used in the lateral ligamentous complex will not work in the deltoid, particularly given the limited vascularity of the degenerated ligament. These ligaments tend to be chronically degenerated and, therefore, will stretch out and eventually fail in standard Brostrom-type reconstructive procedures. Furthermore, unlike lateral ligamentous reconstruction, deltoid ligament reconstruction requires sufficient tension to prevent valgus deformation.[26] Although Hintermann[14] reported good results in acute injuries with the use of suture anchor, which can either be placed proximally or distally, he acknowledges that there is a challenge in patients who have chronic injuries.

### Techniques for Deltoid Ligament Reconstruction

#### Myerson method
First, the group of patients eligible for this type of surgery is examined (see previous discussion of the method and indications for fluoroscopy). Patients in whom the ankle

is in neutral on a weightbearing radiograph but tilt into valgus on stress testing are treated with a deltoid reconstruction (generally in addition to whatever the surgical plan for the ruptured PTT happens to be) (**Figs. 5–11**).

In the group of patients who have a stage IVA rupture with a flexible ankle, a reconstruction will generally succeed. Those who are mobile but require a lot of manipulation to get the ankle into neutral can still be reconstructed; however, one must perform a lateral ankle ligament release and additionally consider slightly weakening the eversion force laterally by transfer of the peroneus brevis into longus. For many years, the senior author has been performing a transfer of the peroneus brevis into the peroneus longus tendon at the level of the calcaneus in conjunction with the reconstruction of a flat foot deformity in which the flexor digitorum longus (FDL) tendon is used to replace the torn PTT. This has the benefit of slightly weakening eversion and simultaneously strengthening first ray plantarflexion.

If, however, the lateral ankle is tight and under fluoroscopy more force is required to maintain a neutral position of the talus before tightening the deltoid reconstruction, the lateral ankle ligaments needs to be released. This can be done through a small anterolateral incision releasing the anterior talofibular ligament off the talus and, if this is not enough, the calcaneofibular ligament through the same incision by peeling it off the calcaneus. This procedure must be done in a stepwise manner by starting slowly with a gentle partial release of the anterior talofibular ligament (ATFL), again checking the stability of the ankle under fluoroscopy and continuing the process until there is little force required to maintain the talus in neutral.

The preferred technique by the senior author has been previously described.[13,26] The principle of the reconstruction is to use a Y-shaped allograft to reconstruct the superficial and the deep portions of the deltoid ligament. The graft length should be at least 20 cm. There are alternative options for preparation of the graft. Generally, the

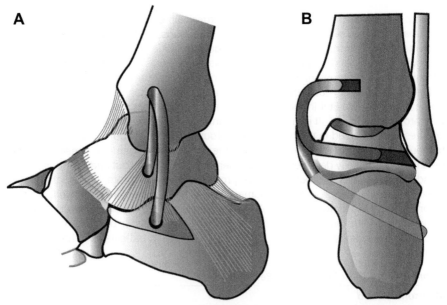

**Fig. 5.** Coronal trajectory of the graft. (*A*) Trajectory in sagittal plane. (*B*) Trajectory in coronal plane.

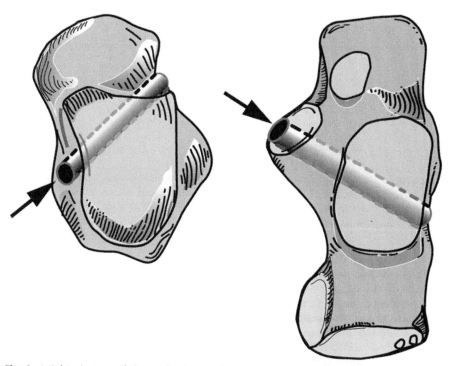

**Fig. 6.** Axial trajectory of the graft. *Arrows* shows entry point and trajectory of graft.

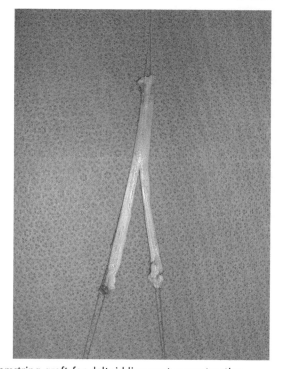

**Fig. 7.** Forked hamstring graft for deltoid ligament reconstruction.

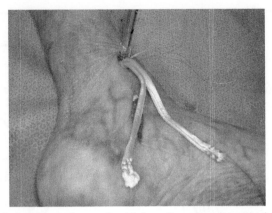

**Fig. 8.** Cadaveric forked hamstring graft with insertion of graft in tibial tunnel.

authors use a hamstring graft, which is far too wide and too long but can be shaped and cut to the appropriate length and then doubled for a double-strand graft. The double ends do not appear as flimsy as a single-strand graft. One end of the graft is split into 2. A stem of about 5 cm is left at the end of the main stem. A hamstring graft is used for reconstruction but any tendon graft may be used. One of the potential problems of using allograft tissue of this type is that the graft tends to stretch out, leading to recurrent medical instability. The authors have recently begun using a hamstring graft and supplementing it with fiber tape or heavy nonabsorbable fiber wire suture. The tape or suture can be woven through the graft, potentially increasing its long-term stability.

The technique involves drilling 3 tunnels into the tibia, talus, and calcaneus. A tibial tunnel is drilled into the medial malleolus and the full tendon inserted and fixed with an interference screw. If the tendon pulls out, then a different technique is used and the tendon is passed obliquely across to the lateral tibia and fixed with a suture button or endobutton (see **Figs. 5–11**).

One limb is then tunneled into the talus. The talar tunnel starts at the medial center of tibiotalar rotation and exits at the lateral junction of the talar dome and neck. This represents the deep portion of the deltoid ligament. The lateral exit point is located by

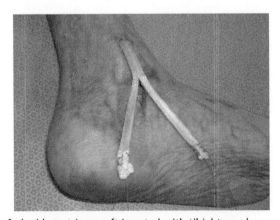

**Fig. 9.** Cadaveric forked hamstring graft inserted with tibial tunnel.

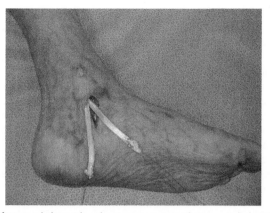

**Fig. 10.** Distal graft passed through subcutaneous tunnel over medial malleolus.

palpation or by a small incision in the lateral neck body junction. The graft is not yet tensioned, which is done at the end of the procedure when both limbs of the graft can be tensioned simultaneously with an interference screw.

The final step is insertion of the second limb into the calcaneus. The tunnel is created along an axis from the sustentaculum talus to a point approximately 1 cm posterior to the calcaneal cuboid joint superior to the peroneal tubercle laterally. The remaining limb of the graft is passed through the calcaneus, representing the superficial part of the native deltoid. The graft is tensioned manually again by pulling on the suture attached to the tip of the graft; pulling it out laterally; and, under maximum tension, securing it medially with an interference screw.

The indications for using this double-strand graft are easier when there is obvious instability. Often, however, clinicians make an error with the diagnosis and find a tear without any instability at the time of surgery. The location of pain is frequently directly under the medical malleolus and there have been times when a diagnosis is made of a spring ligament tear that is later found to be normal but there is a rent in the deltoid. In these cases, it is not clear how aggressive one must be with the

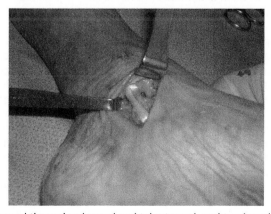

**Fig. 11.** Tendon passed through calcaneal and talar tunnel, and tensioned and secured with 5.5 mm bioabsorbable interference screw.

reconstruction. When the deltoid is chronically torn, the remaining deltoid tissue is thinned out, absent, or frayed beyond any type of repair. In the minor cases, in which the deltoid, both superficial and deep, seems to be intact, but there is a longitudinal full thickness rent in the ligament when probed, there is usually sufficient tissue to perform some type of repair. It is not clear what capacity this ligament has for ligament healing when no longer under constant load with the flat foot. Therefore, the authors have used a medial Brostrom-type procedure for these cases, with an anchor in the medial malleolus and sutures placed so as to slightly imbricate the ligament. The same procedure could be used for a patient who is quite stable on weightbearing radiograph, shows minimal opening under fluoroscopic stress radiograph, and in which there is sufficient tissue to perform this simpler procedure. There are no long-term results on the use of this suture anchor technique and many modifications can, of course, be used to reinforce the medial ankle.

### Postoperative Care

The postoperative protocol includes immediate immobilization in a well-padded plaster splint for 2 weeks. The patient then goes into a boot for 4 weeks but remains nonweightbearing for this time. Further immobilization must continue for another 4 to 6 weeks so that the total period of immobilization is approximately 10 to 12 weeks. The deltoid does not respond nor heal in the same manner as the lateral ligament complex following repair. Physical therapy that includes range of motion, strengthening, and gait training may only start at about 10 to 12 weeks. The ultimate aim is postoperative protocol is to transition to a regular shoe at the 12 weeks.

## PEARLS AND PITFALLS

Although deltoid ligament reconstruction is a legitimate part of correction of flat foot deformity, in patients with stage 4A PTT rupture it should be used in conjunction with other procedures that will help correct the flat foot deformity. The stage IVA deformity may be associated with a rigid or a flexible flat foot deformity and, therefore, either a hindfoot arthrodesis or a reconstruction type of procedure will be performed. Invariably, a gastrocnemius recession must be performed, along with other procedures that supplement either the triple arthrodesis or the hindfoot reconstruction, such as a medial cuneiform osteotomy. If this is used to supplement a triple arthrodesis, the results have been acceptable but not uniformly predictable. This may have something to do with mild, persistent, slight valgus of the ankle at the time of the procedure, inability to completely release the lateral ankle ligaments, or erosive changes in the lateral tibial plafond that allow the ankle to drift back into valgus. These are separate from the increased loads on the medial ankle following a triple arthrodesis.

For this reason, one should consider adding a medial translational osteotomy of the calcaneus at the same time as the hindfoot arthrodesis. This can be done through 1 or 2 lateral incisions, with a generous medial shift of the calcaneus, using the same screw for the calcaneus osteotomy as for the subtalar arthrodesis. When the authors reported on the small group of patients undergoing the double-strand technique for reconstruction, it is likely that we did not completely release laterally, leaving some lateral tension on the ankle, made worse by the stretching out of the hamstring graft (see previous discussion).

One of the problems the authors have encountered with the Y-shaped graft is that the insertion into the medial malleolus may be weak due to osteopenia in this older group of patients. If this occurs, and the graft pulls out, we use an alternative technique (see previous discussion) and, instead of using an interference screw through the medial malleolus, a suture button on the proximal lateral tibia is used, deploying the graft in the same manner but taking advantage of the harder tibial bone to prevent pull out of the graft.

Various nerves may be injured in deltoid ligament reconstruction. When drilling the calcaneal tunnel at the sustentaculum, the tibial is at risk at the lower end of the medial incision. Branches to the sural nerve may also be injured when pulling the calcaneal limb of the graft in the method described by Myerson.[25] Placement of the calcaneal tunnel into the region of the sustentaculum may present a challenge and a guide pin should be used under fluoroscopy to find the correct insertion point on a true lateral radiograph image of the foot. In addition to fracture of the sustentaculum, one must be careful of the flexor hallucis longus (FHL) tendon, which lies immediately under the sustentaculum. The authors generally sweep away the tendon by deep retraction with a periosteal elevator and place the tunnel just deep to the FHL path to avoid tendinitis longus.[14]

## SUMMARY

Deltoid ligament reconstruction allows for joint preservation of the ankle in the setting of patients a triple arthrodesis due to a flat foot deformity. Although the increased forces that may occur in the ankle joint after a triple arthrodesis cannot be eliminated, reconstruction of the ligament will delay and may prevent the onset arthritis. This will allow the patient to maintain mobility of the ankle joint.

## REFERENCES

1. Myerson MS. Adult acquired flatfoot deformity: treatment of rupture of the posterior tibial tendon. Instr Course Lect 1997;46:393–405.
2. Myerson MS. Correction of flat foot deformity in the adult. In: Reconstructive foot and ankle surgery: management of complications. 2nd edition. Philadelphia: Saunders; 2010. p. 201–20.
3. Boss AP, Hintermann B. Anatomical study of the medial ankle ligament complex. Foot Ankle Int 2002;23(6):547–53.
4. Kelikian AS, Sarrafian SK. Sarrafian's anatomy of the foot and ankle: descriptive, topographic, functional. Philadelphia: Wolters Kluwer Health/Lippincott Williams & Wilkins; 2011. p. 176–88.
5. Milner CE, Soames RW. Anatomy of the collateral ligaments of the human ankle joint. Foot Ankle Int 1998;19(11):757–60.
6. Milner CE, Soames RW. The medial collateral ligaments of the human ankle joint: anatomical variations. Foot Ankle Int 1998;19(5):289–92.
7. Campbell KJ, Michalski MP, Wilson KJ, et al. The ligament anatomy of the deltoid complex of the ankle: a qualitative and quantitative anatomical study. J Bone Joint Surg Am 2014;96(8):e62.
8. Harper MC. Deltoid ligament: an anatomical evaluation of function. Foot Ankle 1987;8(1):19–22.
9. Rasmussen O, Kromann-Andersen C, Boe S. Deltoid ligament: Functional analysis of the medial collateral ligamentous apparatus of the ankle joint. Acta Orthop Scand 1983;54:36–44.
10. Earll M, Wayne J, Brodrick C, et al. Contribution of the deltoid ligament to the ankle joint contact characteristics: a cadaver study. Foot Ankle Int 1996;17:317–24.

11. Resnick RB, Jahss MH, Choueka J, et al. Deltoid ligament forces after tibialis posterior tendon rupture: effects of triple arthrodesis and calcaneal displacement osteotomies. Foot Ankle Int 1995;16:14–20.
12. Song SJ, Lee S, O'Malley MJ, et al. Deltoid ligament strain after correction of acquired flatfoot deformity by triple arthrodesis. Foot Ankle Int 2000;21:573–7.
13. Bluman EM, deAsla RJ. Deltoid Ligament Reconstruction. In: Easley M, editor. Operative techniques in foot and ankle surgery. Philadelphia: Lippincott Williams; 2011. p. 867–73.
14. Hintermann B. Medial ankle instability. Foot Ankle Clin 2003;8:723–38.
15. Hintermann B, Valderrabano V, Boss AP, et al. Medial ankle instability an exploratory, prospective study of 52 cases. Am J Sports Med 2004;32:183–90.
16. Tornetta P III. Competence of the deltoid ligament in bimalleolar ankle fractures after medial malleolar fixation. J Bone Joint Surg Am 2000;82A:843–8.
17. Berkes MB, Little MT, Lazaro LE, et al. Malleolar fractures and their ligamentous injury equivalents have similar outcomes in supination-external rotation type IV fractures of the ankle treated by anatomical internal fixation. J Bone Joint Surg Br 2012;94(11):1567–72.
18. Stromsoe K, Hoqevold HE, Skjeldal S, et al. The repair of a ruptured deltoid ligament is not necessary in ankle fractures. J Bone Joint Surg Br 1995;77(6):920–1.
19. Zeegers AV, van der Werken C. Rupture of the deltoid ligament in ankle fractures: should it be repaired? Injury 1989;20(1):39–41.
20. Hsu AR, Lareau CR, Anderson RB. Repair of acute superficial deltoid complex avulsion during ankle fracture fixation in National Football League Players. Foot Ankle Int 2015;36(11):1272–8.
21. Lack W, Phisitkul P, Femino JE. Anatomic deltoid ligament repair with anchor-to-post suture reinforcement: technique tip. Iowa Orthop J 2012;32:227–30.
22. Hintermann B, Knupp M, Pagenstert GI. Deltoid ligament injuries: diagnosis and management. Foot Ankle Clin 2006;11(3):625–37.
23. Haddad SL, Dedhia S, Ren Y, et al. Deltoid ligament reconstruction: a novel technique with biomechanical analysis. Foot Ankle Int 2010;31(7):639–51.
24. Deland JT, de Asla RJ, Segal A. Reconstruction of the chronically failed deltoid ligament: a new technique. Foot Ankle Int 2004;25:795–9.
25. Blumen E, Myerson M. Stage IV posterior tibial tendon rupture. Foot Ankle Clin 2007;12:341–62.
26. Haddad S, Deland J. Mann's Surgery of the foot and ankle. In: Coughlin M, Saltzman C, Anderson R, editors. 9th edition. Elseivier Saunders; 2014. p. 1292–360.

# What to Do with the Spring Ligament

Brian Steginsky, DO, Anand Vora, MD*

## KEYWORDS

- Spring ligament • Calcaneonavicular ligament • Posterior tibial tendon dysfunction
- Flatfoot • Pes planovalgus

## KEY POINTS

- The spring ligament complex is an important static restraint of the medial longitudinal arch of the foot and its failure has been associated with progressive flatfoot deformity.
- Reconstruction of the spring ligament is most appropriate in stage II posterior tibial tendon dysfunction, before severe peritalar subluxation and rigid deformity develops.
- Reconstruction of the spring ligament complex reestablishes a medial soft tissue restraint to minimize talonavicular joint subluxation and mitigate the need for nonanatomic bony procedures that have been associated with complications.
- Although most orthopedic foot and ankle surgeons perform spring ligament reconstruction for stage II deformity, there is still no current consensus regarding the best reconstruction technique.

## INTRODUCTION

The calcaneonavicular ligament, commonly referred to as the spring ligament, is an important static restraint of the medial longitudinal arch. Failure of the spring ligament complex has been implicated in acquired flatfoot deformity.[1] Numerous surgical techniques have been described for the treatment of stage II posterior tibial tendon insufficiency, without a consensus among orthopedic foot and ankle surgeons in regards to the best treatment approach.[2] Reconstruction of the spring ligament is a powerful method of correcting peritalar subluxation and can minimize the need for nonanatomic reconstructive procedures. The role of spring ligament reconstruction is still debated and is the topic of ongoing investigation. This article reviews the pathoanatomy of the spring ligament complex and the potential role of spring

Disclosure Statement: Dr A. Vora is a Consultant for Arthrex. Dr B. Steginsky has nothing to disclose.
Illinois Bone and Joint Institute, 720 Florsheim Drive, Libertyville, IL 60048, USA
* Corresponding author.
E-mail address: dranandvora@gmail.com

ligament reconstruction in acquired flatfoot deformity, and highlights the most current research.

## ANATOMY OF THE SPRING LIGAMENT COMPLEX

The spring ligament complex is a ligamentous structure that extends from the calcaneus to the tarsal navicular. The spring ligament complex supports the head of the talus by resisting plantar and medial talar head subluxation that occurs in more severe acquired flatfoot deformity. The bony and ligamentous structures that suspend and stabilize the talus at the talocalcaneonavicular articulation, including the spring ligament complex, has been collectively referred to as the acetabulum pedis.[3] The structures that form the acetabulum pedis include the anterior and middle articular facets of the calcaneus, the articular facet of the navicular, and the spring ligament complex.

The term spring ligament is a misnomer and has been used inconsistently in the literature to describe various supporting ligamentous and capsular structures of the medial talonavicular articulation.[4,5] Davis and colleagues[4] described two distinct ligamentous bands, the superomedial calcaneonavicular (SMCN) ligament and the inferior calcaneonavicular (ICN) ligament, which have collectively been referred to as the "spring ligament complex." The authors report that the spring ligament complex does not actually possess spring-like properties, but rather functions to provide a sling for the head of the talus.

The SMCN ligament is more than twice as strong as the ICN ligament, with an average load to failure of 665.5 N compared with 291.4 N, respectively.[4] The SMCN ligament is wider, longer, and thicker than the ICN ligament.[4] The origin of the SMCN ligament is from the sustentaclum tali and anterior facet of the calcaneus. The fibers project broadly and assume a concave shape before its insertion at the superior, medial, and inferior articular edge of the navicular.[4] The superficial fibers of the SMCN ligament are flattened by the posterior tibial tendon, which runs immediately adjacent to ligament, and is inspected during surgery with retraction of the tendon. The deep portion of the SMCN ligament contains a fibrocartilage facet that articulates with the plantar-medial aspect of the talar head. The fibrocartilage facet and histologic composition of the SMCN ligament suggests its primary role in load bearing.[4] The ICN ligament lacks a fibrocartilage facet and is primarily subjected to tensile forces.[4] The posterior tibial tendon has distal attachments to the SMCN ligament just proximal to its insertion at the navicular tubercle. The anterior portion of the superficial deltoid ligament also contributes fibers that insert directly onto the superior margin of the SMCN ligament. The distal extent of the SMCN is most frequently injured.[1,6]

The ICN ligament runs plantar and lateral to the SMCN ligament. The origin of the ICN ligament is between the anterior and middle calcaneal facets. The ligament extends medial and distal to its insertion at the inferior cortex of the navicular. The ICN ligament is located directly underneath the talonavicular joint, making it difficult to visualize during surgery.[5] The two bands of the spring ligament complex are demarcated by the routine presence of fat located near the navicular insertion.[3,4]

More recently, Taniguchi and colleagues[3] identified a third ligamentous structure that runs from the notch between the anterior and middle calcaneal articular facets to the navicular tuberosity (**Fig. 1**). The authors coined this structure the "third ligament" and report that it is a distinct part of the spring ligament complex.

The spring ligament complex receives its blood supply from penetrating branches of the medial plantar artery and calcaneal artery.[4] Indirect contributions arise at the sites of its ligamentous attachments to the navicular and sustentaculum tali. The central-third of the spring ligament complex is relatively avascular.

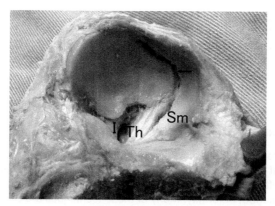

**Fig. 1.** The talus has been excised to demonstrate the anatomy of the acetabulum pedis. The third ligament (Th) runs from the notch between the anterior and middle calcaneal facets to the navicular tuberosity. The orientation of superomedial calcaneonavicular ligament (Sm) and inferior calcaneonavicular ligament (I) is demonstrated. (*From* Taniguchi A, Tanaka Y, Takakura Y, et al. Anatomy of the spring ligament. J Bone Joint Surg Am 2003;85-A(11):2174–8; with permission.)

## PATHOANATOMY

The static soft tissue restraints of the medial longitudinal arch include the spring ligament complex, superficial deltoid ligament, medial talonavicular joint capsule, plantar fascia, and the talocalcaneal ligaments.[7] Deland and coworkers[1] studied the MRI findings of patients with posterior tibial tendon insufficiency to determine the ligaments that were most commonly involved in acquired flatfoot deformity. Several ligaments were found to have pathologic changes on MRI evaluation. However, the spring ligament complex and talocalcaneal interosseous ligament were most frequently implicated. All patients with posterior tibial tendon insufficiency demonstrated some degree of spring ligament complex attenuation on MRI and 74% were diagnosed with a spring ligament tear.

The major dynamic stabilizer of the medial longitudinal arch is the posterior tibial tendon.[8] Functional loss of the posterior tibial tendon transfers stress to the medial ligamentous structures, resulting in progressive attenuation of the soft tissues and subsequent development of an acquired flatfoot deformity.[7–12] Cadaveric studies have determined that posterior tibial tendon insufficiency alone does not result in flatfoot deformity.[9,13] The medial soft tissue structures, including the spring ligament complex, must also fail for deformity to develop. Although tendon transfers are frequently performed to augment the posterior tibial tendon and restore dynamic support to the medial longitudinal arch, these procedures have routinely failed to correct deformity.[11,12,14]

Although posterior tibial tendon dysfunction is the most common cause of flatfoot deformity, traumatic rupture of the spring ligament complex without posterior tibial tendon dysfunction has also been reported to result in flatfoot deformity.[15–17] History of an acute injury should prompt the clinician to consider this diagnosis.

Although the spring ligament complex has been the focus of ligament reconstruction in flatfoot surgery, numerous authors have reported that arch stability is provided by the cumulative effect of several soft tissue restraints.[18–22] In a cadaveric study, Huang and colleagues[23] evaluated the biomechanical effects of progressive ligamentous failure by sequentially dividing the spring ligament complex, plantar fascia, and long and short plantar ligaments. The authors found that the plantar fascia was the most important structure tested, providing approximately 25% of the medial longitudinal arch stiffness. Reeck and colleagues[18] report that the SMCN ligament only supports 10% of ground reactive forces transferred through the acetabulum pedis. However, the orientation and location of the spring ligament complex makes it an important restraint at the talonavicular joint and a critical ligament to recreate in flatfoot reconstructive surgery.

## THE ROLE OF SPRING LIGAMENT RECONSTRUCTION

Johnson and Strom[24] described a staging system to guide the surgical management of posterior tibial tendon dysfunction. Several joint-preserving osteotomies, tendon transfers, and soft tissue reconstructive techniques have been described in the treatment of stage II flatfoot deformity. Many of these techniques are only appropriate for flexible flatfoot deformities. As the medial longitudinal arch continues to collapse, the deformity becomes rigid and fusions become necessary.

The surgical management of stage II posterior tibial tendon dysfunction is one of the most controversial topics among orthopedic foot and ankle surgeons. In 2002, Hiller and Pinney[2] surveyed 128 orthopedic foot and ankle surgeons to inquire about their preferred surgical treatment plan for a healthy and active 62-year-old man with stage II posterior tibial tendon dysfunction. The questionnaire response rate was 81% (104 of 128). Ninety-eight percent (102 of 104) of respondents would perform a soft tissue procedure, of which 53% (55 of 104) would perform a spring ligament repair (**Table 1**). Ninety-seven percent of orthopedic surgeons would perform some type of bony procedure, of which only 12% (12 of 104) reported that they would perform a hindfoot arthrodesis (**Table 2**). Most respondents would use more than one procedure. The most common combination (38%; 39 of 104) included a medial slide calcaneal osteotomy and posterior tibial tendon augmentation.

Concomitant procedures, such as a tendon transfer or calcaneal osteotomy, make it difficult to quantify the exact benefit of an in vivo spring ligament reconstruction. However, several authors have demonstrated the corrective power of an isolated spring ligament reconstruction in a cadaveric flatfoot model.[25–27] Reconstruction of the spring ligament, when used as an adjunct procedure in flatfoot reconstruction, may

| Table 1 Soft tissue procedures most frequently performed for stage II posterior tibial tendon dysfunction | |
|---|---|
| **Soft Tissue Procedure** | **Number (n = 104) (%)** |
| Posterior tibial tendon augmentation | 98 (94) |
| FDL tendon transfer | 89 (86) |
| FHL tendon transfer | 9 (9) |
| Spring ligament repair | 55 (53) |
| Deltoid ligament repair | 7 (7) |
| Equinas contracture correction | 73 (70) |
| No soft tissue procedure | 2 (2) |

Academic orthopedic foot and ankle surgeons were surveyed in 2002 (n = 128). The questionnaire response rate was 81%.

*Abbreviations:* FDL, flexor digitorum longus; FHL, flexor hallucis longus.

*Data from* Hiller L, Pinney SJ. Surgical treatment of acquired flatfoot deformity: what is the state of practice among academic foot and ankle surgeons in 2002? Foot Ankle Int 2003;24(9):701–5.

| Table 2 Bony procedures most frequently performed for stage II posterior tibial tendon dysfunction | |
|---|---|
| **Bony Procedures** | **Number (n = 104) (%)** |
| Medializing calcaneal osteotomy | 76 (73) |
| Lateral column lengthening | 43 (41) |
|   Evans procedures | 21 (20) |
|   Calcaneocuboid arthrodesis | 22 (21) |
| Medial column stabilization | 16 (15) |
|   Navicular-cuneiform arthrodesis | 4 (4) |
|   First tarsometatarsal arthrodesis | 9 (9) |
|   Both | 3 (3) |
| Hindfoot arthrodesis | 12 (12) |
|   Subtalar | 9 (9) |
|   Triple | 1 (1) |
|   Talonavicular | 2 (2) |
| No bony procedure | 3 (3) |

Academic orthopedic foot and ankle surgeons were surveyed in 2002 (n = 128). The questionnaire response rate was 81%.

*Data from* Hiller L, Pinney SJ. Surgical treatment of acquired flatfoot deformity: what is the state of practice among academic foot and ankle surgeons in 2002? Foot Ankle Int 2003;24(9):701–5.

also obviate lateral column lengthening, subtalar arthrodesis, and midfoot fusions. Although nonanatomic bony procedures are often used to improve alignment, they have also been associated with increased pain, stiffness, and adjacent joint arthritis.[22]

Indications for spring ligament reconstruction are not well defined and there is a lack of consensus among orthopedic foot and ankle surgeons. Deland[22] recommends spring ligament reconstruction when there is significant residual deformity at the talonavicular joint after performing a lateral column lengthening and medial displacement calcaneal osteotomy. If intraoperative fluoroscopic evaluation reveals greater than 30° of talonavicular uncoverage on the anteroposterior image or more than 10° of plantar sag on the lateral image, spring ligament reconstruction should be considered.[28] Flatfoot deformity is best treated before severe deformity develops (stage IIB).[5] Other authors argue that spring ligament reconstruction may obviate nonanatomic reconstructive procedures, including lateral column lengthening.[29]

The most common bony procedure in stage II posterior tibial tendon dysfunction is a medial displacement calcaneal osteotomy, which is performed by 73% of orthopedic foot and ankle surgeons.[2] Otis and colleagues[30] performed a cadaveric study to investigate the effect of a medial displacement calcaneal osteotomy on the length of the spring ligament complex. Although elongation of the spring ligament occurred with simulated weight bearing, the medial displacement calcaneal osteotomy resulted in a relative shortening of the ligament when compared with control subjects. The reduced strain and relative shortening of the spring ligament complex highlights the protective effect of the medial displacement calcaneal osteotomy. Other studies have also demonstrated the protective effects of a medial slide calcaneal osteotomy on the medial longitudinal arch, including the superficial deltoid ligament.[31] We advocate performing a medial displacement calcaneal osteotomy to achieve hindfoot correction and protect the spring ligament reconstruction.

Similarly, lateral column lengthening would be expected to protect the spring ligament complex by reducing the talonavicular joint and shifting the forefoot contact point to a more medial position. However, Otis and colleagues[32] reported that lateral column lengthening does not reduce strain on the spring ligament complex or offer any protective effect. Lateral column lengthening is a nonanatomic technique that has been associated with increased plantar pressures and lateral foot pain.[33] Other complications of lateral column lengthening include nonunion and fifth metatarsal stress fractures.[34,35] Lateral column lengthening may be suitable for more severe forefoot abduction deformities. We believe that spring ligament reconstruction is a tremendously powerful technique that may minimize dependence on nonanatomic lateral column lengthening procedures that have been associated with complications.

## DIAGNOSIS

There is no reliable clinical test to detect spring ligament pathology. The diagnosis depends on MRI evaluation and direct intraoperative inspection. The sensitivity of spring ligament insufficiency on MRI is reported to range from 55% to 77%, whereas specificity is 100%.[36] MRI findings consistent with spring ligament insufficiency include increased signal changes on T2-weighted sequences associated with thickening (>5 mm) or thinning (<2 mm) of the SMCN ligament.[6,37]

## REPAIR OR RECONSTRUCTION?

Reconstruction of the spring ligament complex is favored over direct repair.[5] Failure of the spring ligament complex in the setting of posterior tibial tendon insufficiency is often the result of a degenerative process, in which the native tissues of the spring ligament complex become attenuated and incapable of holding a repair. The robust graft tissue used in a reconstructive procedure is more likely to resist the strain at the talonavicular joint and maintain correction. Spring ligament reconstruction has been performed using the superficial deltoid ligament, peroneus longus tendon, split anterior tibial tendon, and flexor hallucis longus tendon. Tendon harvest is associated with some degree of patient morbidity and loss of strength. Acevedo and Vora[29] introduced the technique of direct spring ligament repair with polyethylene fiber tape augmentation, minimizing the need to perform reconstructive techniques that rely on tendon harvest. Direct repair of the spring ligament complex may also be suitable in the scenario of an acute or subacute ligamentous injury, before the soft tissues become attenuated.[15,16]

## CADAVERIC STUDIES

Most knowledge regarding the spring ligament complex and its implication in flatfoot deformity has originated from cadaveric studies. The confounding effect of concomitant procedures performed at the time of spring ligament reconstruction has been a major limitation of many clinical studies. Cadaveric flatfoot models provide the opportunity to investigate isolated spring ligament reconstruction and delineate its potential use for in vivo reconstructive surgery.

Deland and colleagues[20] created one of the first cadaveric flatfoot models by releasing the spring ligament complex, medial aspect of the calcaneocuboid joint, and long plantar ligament. The authors noted a mild flatfoot deformity after initial ligamentous release. Severe flatfoot deformity was recreated by additional release of the plantar fascia, superficial deltoid ligament, capsule of the medial subtalar joint, and talocalcaneal interosseous ligament. Significant talonavicular joint subluxation ensued following release of the static soft tissue restraints. Radiographic measurement of the talonavicular angle revealed an average change of 34.6° (anteroposterior) and 18.1°

(lateral) compared with an intact cadaveric foot. Isolated release of the posterior tibial tendon did not result in any radiographic abnormality.

The authors harvested a deltoid ligament bone-block graft from the medial malleolus to reconstruct the spring ligament complex. The superficial deltoid ligament was left intact at its insertion to the sustentaculum tali. The bone-block was fixed to the medial cortex of the navicular after reducing the deformity and while maintaining appropriate tension on the graft. Reconstruction of the spring ligament brought the talonavicular angle to within a couple degrees of the intact control specimen on the lateral and anteroposterior radiographs. Bone-block fractures occurred in two specimens (20%), but did not result in graft failure. Preservation of the deep deltoid ligament prevented postreconstruction tibiotalar valgus instability. The authors expressed concern about the robustness of the deltoid reconstruction technique and have since abandoned its use in exchange for Achilles tendon allograft.

Thordarson and colleagues[21] used a cadaveric flatfoot model to compare four different techniques for flatfoot reconstruction. The authors divided the spring ligament, talonavicular joint capsule, anteromedial subtalar joint capsule, and plantar fascia to recreate a flatfoot deformity. The peroneus longus tendon was transected proximal to the superior peroneal retinaculum, leaving its distal insertion intact at the base of the first metatarsal and medial cuneiform. The tendon was delivered through an incision on the medial aspect of the foot and subsequently passed medial to lateral through a bone tunnel in the calcaneus. The flatfoot deformity was reduced and the peroneus longus tendon was secured with a screw and washer to the lateral wall of the calcaneus. Flatfoot reconstruction was also repeated using a split anterior tibial tendon graft and Achilles tendon allograft. After spring ligament reconstruction, each specimen was sequentially loaded with increasing weight and displacement across the medial longitudinal arch was tracked by measuring the angular relationship between the first metatarsal and talus. When compared with the other reconstruction methods, the peroneus longus tendon tenodesis provided greater correction of the deformity in the sagittal and transverse planes across all loads, except in the transverse plane at a maximum load of 700 N.[21] The other three techniques performed poorly in comparison, demonstrating premature graft failure and loss of alignment at much less load. The peroneus longus tendon is a major contributor to forefoot abduction and sacrifice of the tendon may neutralize its deforming forces on the midfoot, offering a secondary advantage with its use. Potential disadvantages of a peroneus longus tendon autograft include donor site morbidity and loss of dynamic first-ray plantar flexion. Thordarson and colleagues[21] was the first to describe the peroneus longus tendon technique for spring ligament reconstruction.

Choi and colleagues[27] compared multiple different techniques of spring ligament reconstruction also using the peroneus longus tendon. The peroneus longus tendon was harvested and delivered through an incision on the medial aspect of the midfoot as previously described by Thordarson and colleagues.[21] The superomedial and plantar bands of the spring ligament complex were recreated by passing the free-end of the graft from medial to lateral through an anterior calcaneal bone tunnel, then passing the graft back from lateral to medial through a slightly more posterior calcaneal bone tunnel. Lastly, the free-end of the graft was passed from dorsal to plantar through the navicular bone tunnel and secured to itself with nonabsorbable suture. The combined superomedial and plantar reconstruction technique performed better during cadaveric load testing compared with reconstruction of either the superomedial or plantar band alone. The talonavicular abduction deformity in the flatfoot model, after ligamentous release, was 9.1° ± 8.1° in the coronal plane. The flatfoot deformity in the present study was mild in comparison with previous cadaveric flatfoot models.[20,21] The combined superomedial and plantar reconstruction resulted in a 1.0° overcorrection (adduction) at the talonavicular joint in the coronal plane. Subtalar joint alignment corrected from 3.1° of eversion in the flatfoot model to 0.4° of inversion after combined reconstruction of the superomedial and plantar bands of the spring ligament. The authors advocate anatomic reconstruction of the spring ligament complex, because the combined reconstruction technique more closely resembles the anatomy and physiology of an intact foot.

In contrast, Baxter and colleagues[25] reported that nonanatomic ligamentous reconstruction of the medial longitudinal arch resulted in greater correction of the deformity compared with an anatomic spring ligament reconstruction. The authors tested several reconstruction methods by fixing the graft in different positions to recreate the various static soft tissue restraints of the medial longitudinal arch. Combined reconstruction of the superficial deltoid ligament and superomedial spring ligament resulted in two to four times greater deformity correction compared with an anatomic reconstruction of the spring ligament alone. Surprisingly, anatomic spring ligament reconstruction provided the least amount of talonavicular and hindfoot correction under loaded conditions when compared with the other reconstructive techniques. The results reinforce the findings of several previous studies, reminding us that the spring ligament complex is an important structure, but other ligaments are critical to the structural integrity of the medial longitudinal arch.[18–22]

Tan and colleagues[26] created a severe flatfoot deformity in a cadaveric model by sectioning several medial ligamentous structures and capsule, including the spring ligament complex. The cadaveric specimens were loaded before ligament sectioning (intact foot), after ligament sectioning (flatfoot), and following reconstruction with a split anterior tibial tendon graft spanning from the neck of the talus to the medial cuneiform. Radiographic parameters of the intact foot, flatfoot, and reconstructed foot were recorded for comparison. Reconstruction of the static medial ligamentous complex resulted in a significant improvement in the talus-first metatarsal angle on the anteroposterior and lateral radiographs, and an increase in the medial cuneiform height in comparison with the flatfoot model.

## CLINICAL OUTCOMES

To our knowledge, there have not been any clinical studies that evaluate the efficacy of isolated spring ligament reconstruction. Flatfoot reconstruction often requires a combination of procedures to adequately realign the foot, making it difficult to evaluate the effectiveness of any single technique. The results of the following clinical studies must be interpreted with this in mind.

Goldner and colleagues[10] reported on the clinical outcomes of nine patients with progressive flatfoot deformity secondary to traumatic rupture or degeneration of the posterior tibial tendon. The spring ligament complex was found to be elongated and incompetent in all patients. The fibers of the spring ligament complex and anterior extent of the superficial deltoid ligament were elevated in a proximal-to-distal fashion. The distal-based soft tissue flap was left intact at its insertion on the navicular. Deformity at the talonavicular joint was corrected with proximal advancement of the soft tissue flap. Tendon transfers and plication of the posterior tibial tendon alone was insufficient to restore the longitudinal arch of the foot. The authors performed advancement of the spring ligament to achieve an "anatomic and functional result [with] essentially a normal foot."

Williams and colleagues[28] reported on 13 patients who had spring ligament reconstruction using peroneus longus tendon autograft. All patients were diagnosed with stage IIb posterior tibial tendon dysfunction. Spring ligament reconstruction was performed in patients with persistent talonavicular abduction (>30°) or plantar talonavicular sag (>10°) after fixation of all bony osteotomies. The peroneus longus tendon autograft was harvested and delivered through a medial incision on the foot as previously described by Thordarson and coworkers.[21] The proximal end of the graft was passed from dorsal to plantar through the navicular bone tunnel drilled for the flexor digitorum longus tendon transfer. The free end of the graft was anchored at different positions proximally, which were chosen based on the predominant type of deformity present at the talonavicular joint. The graft was anchored to the calcaneus if plantar sag was the principal deformity. However, the graft was anchored to the medial malleolus if the predominant deformity was talonavicular abduction. A total of 11 of the 13 patients were reported to have excellent functional outcomes at an average of 8.9 years follow-up. The average postoperative American Orthopedic Foot and Ankle Society (AOFAS) score was 90.3, which represents significant improvement from the average preoperative score of 43.1. However, AOFAS scores must be interpreted with caution because data supporting its validity are still lacking. Significant improvement was also seen on several radiographic parameters including the first tarsometatarsal angle, talonavicular coverage angle, lateral calcaneal pitch, and lateral talonavicular angle. A total of 12 of the 13 patients exhibited full eversion strength on postoperative clinical examination. The outcomes were comparable with historical control subjects that had lateral column lengthening without spring ligament reconstruction.[28,38] The authors conclude that spring ligament reconstruction is appropriate for severe flexible flatfoot deformities with persistent talonavicular deformity, which previously would have been treated with a triple arthrodesis.

Lee and Yi[39] used the flexor hallucis longus tendon to reconstruct the spring ligament in 23 patients with flatfoot deformity. The flexor hallucis longus tendon was transected at the metatarsophalangeal (MTP) joint and passed plantar to dorsal through the medial cuneiform, dorsal to plantar through the navicular, and medial to lateral through the sustentaculum tali. The technique reestablishes the static support of the spring ligament complex and the dynamic function of the posterior tibial tendon, eliminating the need for a flexor digitorum longus tendon transfer. At 8.2-month follow-up the average AOFAS score was 86.4, which was an improvement from the mean preoperative score of 72.6. Radiographic alignment also seemed to improve with surgery.

Acevedo and Vora[29] described an anatomic spring ligament reconstruction technique using polyethylene fiber tape. Direct repair of the native spring ligament was performed before fiber tape augmentation. The authors used a fiber tape construct (Arthrex, Naples, FL) to recreate the superomedial and inferior bands of the spring ligament and augment the soft tissue repair (**Fig. 2**). The preloaded anchor was placed into the sustentaculum tali, taking care to protect the flexor hallucis longus tendon and neurovascular bundle. The superomedial band of the spring ligament was recreated by advancing a limb of the fiber tape from dorsal to plantar through the navicular tunnel. The inferomedial band of the spring ligament was replicated by advancing the other limb of the fiber tape from plantar to dorsal through the navicular tunnel (passed with the flexor digitorum longus tendon). The distal construct was secured to the navicular with a biotenodesis screw. The authors successfully performed this technique in 26 patients with only one radiographic failure and partial recurrence of deformity. All patients had a flexor digitorum longus tendon transfer, 25 patients had a medializing calcaneal osteotomy, 11 patients had a gastrocnemius recession, 10 patients had a medial cuneiform opening wedge osteotomy, four patients had a first tarsometatarsal fusion, and two patients had a lateral column lengthening calcaneal osteotomy. The authors noted a greater improvement in foot alignment than would

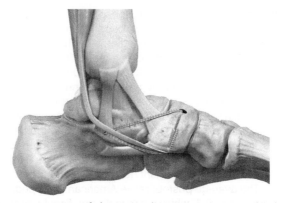

**Fig. 2.** Anatomic reconstruction of the spring ligament using a preloaded suture anchor placed into the sustentaculum tali. The suture limbs and flexor digitorum longus tendon are passed through the navicular tunnel and secured with a biotenodesis screw. (*From* Acevedo J, Vora A. Anatomical reconstruction of the spring ligament complex: "internal brace" augmentation. Foot Ankle Spec 2013;6(6):441–5; with permission.)

otherwise be expected with a flexor digitorum longus tendon transfer and medializing calcaneal osteotomy alone. It was concluded that fiber tape augmentation and direct spring ligament repair can provide substantial corrective power, mitigating the need for nonanatomic reconstructive procedures including lateral column lengthening and subtalar arthrodesis.

Palmanovich and coworkers[40] performed a direct repair of the spring ligament using nonabsorbable suture. Fiber tape (Arthrex) was passed in a figure-of-eight fashion from a drill hole in the navicular tuberosity to a drill hole in the sustentaculum tali. The tails of the fiber tape were then anchored to the medial malleolus to reconstruct the anterior deltoid ligament fibers. Patient outcomes were not reported.

Gazdag and Cracchiolo[41] reported on 22 patients with posterior tibial tendon dysfunction, of which 18 patients were identified with spring ligament pathology. The authors proposed a classification system for spring ligament pathology (**Table 3**). Direct suture repair was performed for all seven patients that had a spring ligament tear without evidence of tissue laxity or attenuation (grade I). Eleven patients were identified with grade 2 or 3 spring ligament pathology. A total of 5 of the 11 patients had spring ligament repair and augmentation with the distal stump of the posterior tibial tendon or superficial deltoid ligament. A total of 6 of the 11 patients had reconstruction of the spring ligament with a split anterior tibial tendon graft anchored to the sustentaculum tali. Seventy-eight percent of patients (14 of 18) who underwent

| Table 3 | |
|---|---|
| **Grading system for spring ligament pathology** | |
| **Grade** | **Spring Ligament Pathology** |
| 1 | Mid-substance tear or insertional tear, without attenuation or laxity |
| 2 | Attenuated ligament, with or without a tear |
| 3 | Complete rupture |

*Data from* Gazdag AR, Cracchiolo A. Rupture of the posterior tibial tendon. Evaluation of injury of the spring ligament and clinical assessment of tendon transfer and ligament repair. J Bone Joint Surg Am 1997;79(5):675–81.

repair of the spring ligament complex had an excellent clinical outcome, reporting a dramatic relief in pain without any limitations in daily recreational activities. However, deformity correction was disappointing. All patients who had spring ligament repair continued to have significant deformity on postoperative radiographic and clinical examination. Bony realignment procedures were not performed in the study. The results highlight the potential limitations of isolated soft tissue procedures in severe flatfoot deformity correction.

## SUMMARY

Although several procedures have been described for the treatment of stage II posterior tibial tendon dysfunction, there is currently no common consensus among orthopedic surgeons regarding the best treatment plan.[2] Tendon transfers and calcaneal osteotomies are performed by most orthopedic foot and ankle surgeons; however, these procedures fail to recreate the important ligamentous structures of the medial longitudinal arch. Attenuation of the medial ligamentous structures, including the spring ligament complex, results in progressive flatfoot deformity. Reconstruction of the spring ligament complex recreates a soft tissue buttress to minimize talonavicular joint subluxation and mitigate the need for nonanatomic bony procedures that have been associated with complications. An interest in spring ligament reconstruction has evolved over the last two decades, with a potential for soft tissue reconstruction to provide an alternative pathway to medial arch restoration with more reliable and satisfying outcomes.

Multiple techniques for spring ligament reconstruction, anatomic and nonanatomic, have been described. There has been paucity in clinical outcome data to suggest the superiority of any single spring ligament reconstruction technique. Spring ligament reconstruction, regardless of the technique, can lend some degree of deformity correction at the talonavicular joint. Spring ligament reconstruction is most advantageous in the early stages of flatfoot deformity, while the foot is supple and peritalar subluxation is contained. Although some authors perform spring ligament reconstruction only after bony corrections have failed, we maintain that spring ligament reconstruction is a joint- and motion-preserving technique that can minimize dependence on nonanatomic bony procedures, particularly lateral column lengthening.

The literature on spring ligament reconstruction has been limited to level IV evidence and expert opinions. We are not aware of any high-level evidence to support or refute the use of spring ligament reconstruction. Despite these facts, more than 50% of orthopedic foot and ankle surgeons repair the spring ligament complex in stage II posterior tibial tendon dysfunction.[2] Spring ligament repair is more commonly performed than lateral column lengthening or hindfoot/medial column arthrodesis, which is a further testament of its utility in the surgical treatment of flatfoot deformity.[2] Although an understanding of the spring ligament complex and its contribution to medial arch stability has grown, there is not yet a unanimously accepted technique that has consistently demonstrated satisfactory outcomes. Future studies must report patient functional outcomes using validated scoring systems, account for the confounding effects of concomitant procedures, and demonstrate longevity in spring ligament reconstruction.

## REFERENCES

1. Deland JT, de Asla RJ, Sung IH, et al. Posterior tibial tendon insufficiency: which ligaments are involved? Foot Ankle Int 2005;26(6):427–35.

2. Hiller L, Pinney SJ. Surgical treatment of acquired flatfoot deformity: what is the state of practice among academic foot and ankle surgeons in 2002? Foot Ankle Int 2003;24(9):701–5.

3. Taniguchi A, Tanaka Y, Takakura Y, et al. Anatomy of the spring ligament. J Bone Joint Surg Am 2003;85-A(11):2174–8.

4. Davis WH, Sobel M, DiCarlo EF, et al. Gross, histological, and microvascular anatomy and biomechanical testing of the spring ligament complex. Foot Ankle Int 1996;17(2):95–102.

5. Deland JT. The adult acquired flatfoot and spring ligament complex. Pathology and implications for treatment. Foot Ankle Clin 2001;6(1):129–35.

6. Mengiardi B, Pinto C, Zanetti M. Spring ligament complex and posterior tibial tendon: MR anatomy and findings in acquired adult flatfoot deformity. Semin Musculoskelet Radiol 2016;20(1):104–15.

7. Sitler DF, Bell SJ. Soft tissue procedures. Foot Ankle Clin 2003;8(3):503–20.

8. Van Boerum DH, Sangeorzan BJ. Biomechanics and pathophysiology of flat foot. Foot Ankle Clin 2003;8(3):419–30.

9. Niki H, Ching RP, Kiser P, et al. The effect of posterior tibial tendon dysfunction on hindfoot kinematics. Foot Ankle Int 2001;22(4):292–300.

10. Goldner JL, Keats PK, Bassett FH, et al. Progressive talipes equinovalgus due to trauma or degeneration of the posterior tibial tendon and medial plantar ligaments. Orthop Clin North Am 1974;5(1):39–51.

11. Mann RA, Thompson FM. Rupture of the posterior tibial tendon causing flat foot. Surgical treatment. J Bone Joint Surg Am 1985;67(4):556–61.

12. Funk DA, Cass JR, Johnson KA. Acquired adult flat foot secondary to posterior tibial-tendon pathology. J Bone Joint Surg Am 1986;68(1):95–102.

13. Jennings MM, Christensen JC. The effects of sectioning the spring ligament on rearfoot stability and posterior tibial tendon efficiency. J Foot Ankle Surg 2008; 47(3):219–24.

14. Deland JT. Posterior tibial tendon insufficiency: soft-tissue reconstruction. Oper Tech Orthop 1992;2(3):157–61.

15. Tryfonidis M, Jackson W, Mansour R, et al. Acquired adult flat foot due to isolated plantar calcaneonavicular (spring) ligament insufficiency with a normal tibialis posterior tendon. Foot Ankle Surg 2008;14(2):89–95.

16. Borton DC, Saxby TS. Tear of the plantar calcaneonavicular (spring) ligament causing flatfoot. A case report. J Bone Joint Surg Br 1997;79(4):641–3.

17. Weerts B, Warmerdam PE, Faber FWM. Isolated spring ligament rupture causing acute flatfoot deformity: case report. Foot Ankle Int 2012;33(2):148–50.

18. Reeck J, Felten N, McCormack AP, et al. Support of the talus: a biomechanical investigation of the contributions of the talonavicular and talocalcaneal joints, and the superomedial calcaneonavicular ligament. Foot Ankle Int 1998;19(10): 674–82.

19. Kitaoka HB, Ahn TK, Luo ZP, et al. Stability of the arch of the foot. Foot Ankle Int 1997;18(10):644–8.

20. Deland JT, Arnoczky SP, Thompson FM. Adult acquired flatfoot deformity at the talonavicular joint: reconstruction of the spring ligament in an in vitro model. Foot Ankle 1992;13(6):327–32.

21. Thordarson DB, Schmotzer H, Chon J. Reconstruction with tenodesis in an adult flatfoot model. A biomechanical evaluation of four methods. J Bone Joint Surg Am 1995;77(10):1557–64.

22. Deland JT. Spring ligament complex and flatfoot deformity: curse or blessing? Foot Ankle Int 2012;33(3):239–43.

23. Huang CK, Kitaoka HB, An KN, et al. Biomechanical evaluation of longitudinal arch stability. Foot Ankle 1993;14(6):353–7.
24. Johnson KA, Strom DE. Tibialis posterior tendon dysfunction. Clin Orthop Relat Res 1989;(239):196–206.
25. Baxter JR, LaMothe JM, Walls RJ, et al. Reconstruction of the medial talonavicular joint in simulated flatfoot deformity. Foot Ankle Int 2015;36(4):424–9.
26. Tan GJ, Kadakia AR, Ruberte Thiele RA, et al. Novel reconstruction of a static medial ligamentous complex in a flatfoot model. Foot Ankle Int 2010;31(8): 695–700.
27. Choi K, Lee S, Otis JC, et al. Anatomical reconstruction of the spring ligament using peroneus longus tendon graft. Foot Ankle Int 2003;24(5):430–6.
28. Williams BR, Ellis SJ, Deyer TW, et al. Reconstruction of the spring ligament using a peroneus longus autograft tendon transfer. Foot Ankle Int 2010;31(7):567–77.
29. Acevedo J, Vora A. Anatomical reconstruction of the spring ligament complex: "internal brace" augmentation. Foot Ankle Spec 2013;6(6):441–5.
30. Otis JC, Deland JT, Kenneally S, et al. Medial arch strain after medial displacement calcaneal osteotomy: an in vitro study. Foot Ankle Int 1999;20(4):222–6.
31. Resnick RB, Jahss MH, Choueka J, et al. Deltoid ligament forces after tibialis posterior tendon rupture: effects of triple arthrodesis and calcaneal displacement osteotomies. Foot Ankle Int 1995;16(1):14–20.
32. Otis JC, Deland JT, Kenneally S. Medial arch strain after lateral column lengthening: an in vitro study. Foot Ankle Int 1999;20(12):797–802.
33. Ellis SJ, Yu JC, Johnson AH, et al. Plantar pressures in patients with and without lateral foot pain after lateral column lengthening. J Bone Joint Surg Am 2010; 92(1):81–91.
34. van der Krans A, Louwerens JW, Anderson P. Adult acquired flexible flatfoot, treated by calcaneo-cuboid distraction arthrodesis, posterior tibial tendon augmentation, and percutaneous Achilles tendon lengthening: a prospective outcome study of 20 patients. Acta Orthop 2006;77(1):156–63.
35. Davitt JS, Morgan JM. Stress fracture of the fifth metatarsal after Evans' calcaneal osteotomy: a report of two cases. Foot Ankle Int 1998;19(10):710–2.
36. Yao L, Gentili A, Cracchiolo A. MR imaging findings in spring ligament insufficiency. Skeletal Radiol 1999;28(5):245–50.
37. Williams G, Widnall J, Evans P, et al. MRI features most often associated with surgically proven tears of the spring ligament complex. Skeletal Radiol 2013;42(7): 969–73.
38. Toolan BC, Sangeorzan BJ, Hansen ST Jr. Complex reconstruction for the treatment of dorsolateral peritalar subluxation of the foot. Early results after distraction arthrodesis of the calcaneocuboid joint in conjunction with stabilization of, and transfer of the flexor digitorum longus tendon to, the midfoot to treat acquired pes planovalgus in adults. J Bone Joint Surg Am 1999;81(11):1545–60.
39. Lee WC, Yi Y. Spring ligament reconstruction using the autogenous flexor hallucis longus tendon. Orthopedics 2014;37(7):467–71.
40. Palmanovich E, Shabat S, Brin YS, et al. Anatomic reconstruction technique for a plantar calcaneonavicular (spring) ligament tear. J Foot Ankle Surg 2015;54(6): 1124–6.
41. Gazdag AR, Cracchiolo A. Rupture of the posterior tibial tendon. Evaluation of injury of the spring ligament and clinical assessment of tendon transfer and ligament repair. J Bone Joint Surg Am 1997;79(5):675–81.

# Naviculocuneiform Sag in the Acquired Flatfoot
## What to Do

Joshua A. Metzl, MD

## KEYWORDS

• Flatfoot • Pes planus • Naviculocuneiform sag • Medial column instability

## KEY POINTS

- No single procedure is enough to address the complexity of the adult acquired flatfoot deformity.
- Careful physical evaluation and weight-bearing radiographs are required to form a comprehensive surgical plan.
- Sag at the naviculocuneiform (NC) joint represents an important aspect of the flatfoot deformity.
- Failure to address medial column instability could lead to continued deformity and poor patient outcomes.
- Whether in combination with other procedures or in isolation, NC fusion and Cotton osteotomy are important pieces of the armamentarium to address all aspects of the flatfoot deformity.

## INTRODUCTION

Medial column collapse in the adult acquired flatfoot is a complex problem with several solutions. The typical flatfoot patient complains of medial or subfibular hindfoot pain with progressive planovalgus deformity. The posterior tibial tendon (PTT), along with the spring ligament complex, provides the structural integrity of the medial ankle. Failure of these structures can lead to collapse of the medial column through the first tarsometatarsal (TMT) joint, naviculocuneiform (NC) joint, or talonavicular (TN) joint.[1]

Physical examination helps to clarify the severity of PTT dysfunction (PTTD). In stage I PTTD, the patient can perform a single limb heel rise with some discomfort, but minimal or no deformity. In stage II, the PTT becomes more diseased and the patient cannot perform a single limb heel rise. The hindfoot valgus is correctable, but residual forefoot varus can sometimes be appreciated (**Fig. 1**). Stage III disease is characterized by a rigid flatfoot that is not passively correctable to neutral. The patient cannot perform a single limb heel rise.

Disclosure: Dr J.A. Metzl is a consultant for Arthrex.
Department of Orthopaedics, UC Health Steadman Hawkins Clinic Denver, 8200 East Belleview Avenue Suite 615, Greenwood Village, CO 80111, USA
E-mail address: joshmetzl@gmail.com

Foot Ankle Clin N Am 22 (2017) 529–544
http://dx.doi.org/10.1016/j.fcl.2017.04.007
**foot.theclinics.com**

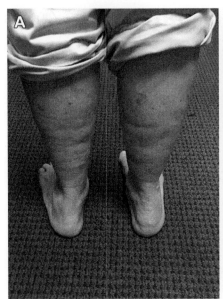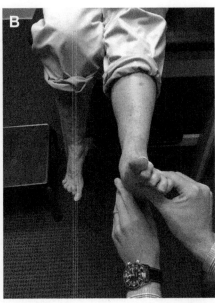

**Fig. 1.** (A) Asymmetric heel valgus on the left side, typical of a patient with PTTD. (B) Residual forefoot varus after correction of hindfoot valgus seen in type IIB flatfoot. Forefoot varus after correction of hindfoot valgus is an excellent indication for a Cotton osteotomy.

Radiographic evaluation of the flatfoot helps to quantify the severity of the problem and to guide treatment. Standing plain films can demonstrate relative shortening of the lateral column compared with the medial column. The TN joint can be 3 to 5 mm shorter than the calcaneocuboid (CC) joint on an anteroposterior (AP) radiograph, as compared with the typical parallel relationship in a normal radiograph. Forefoot abduction is assessed on standing plain films by the coverage of the TN joint. Some surgeons would consider adding a lateral column (ie, lateral column lengthening or distraction CC fusion) procedure with TN uncoverage greater than 50%. Meary's angle is measured on the lateral radiograph and is formed by the intersection of a line drawn down the longitudinal axis of the talus and the first metatarsal. A measurement of less than 30° is considered severe whereas a measurement of 15 to 30° is moderate pes planus.[2] The calcaneal pitch measures the angle between plantar aspect of the calcaneus and the ground. Normal is considered 10 to 30° and less than 10° is considered planus.

The weight-bearing lateral radiograph is the most important study for evaluation of the competence of the medial column. Careful examination of the TN, NC, and TMT joints is required for full evaluation of pes planus deformity. Plantar gapping at the first TMT joint may be indicative of a hypermobile first ray.[1,3] Sag at the NC joint, degenerative changes at the NC joint, or both can be appreciated as well. These findings may be used to guide surgical treatment.

In patients with an apex of deformity at the NC joint, the reverse Coleman block test can also be used to identify if arthrodesis or Cotton osteotomy is indicated.[4] The patient with heel valgus and sag at the NC joint on a standing lateral radiograph is asked to place the first metatarsal on a radiolucent block until the heel valgus is corrected to neutral. Repeat plain films are then obtained. If the NC sag persists, even with correction of hindfoot valgus, then strong consideration should be given to addressing the medial column during surgery.

Recently, the medial arch sag angle (MASA) has been described as a technique to evaluate the contribution of midfoot deformity to pes planus. To evaluate MASA, a line is drawn along the articular surface of the navicular and a second line is drawn parallel to the first TMT joint on a lateral radiograph. The angle where these lines intersect is the MASA.[5]

Treatment of PTTD has many options, including operative and nonoperative. Nonsurgical options include orthotics, physical therapy, and boot or cast immobilization. If these measures fail, surgery may be warranted. Surgical options include tendon debridements, tendon transfers, osteotomies, fusions, or a mixture of these procedures. The mainstay of treatment of the diseased PTT is flexor digitorum longus (FDL) transfer to the navicular. This procedure is sometimes combined with an imbrication of the spring ligament,[6] and a gastrocnemius recession. In most cases of adult acquired flatfoot deformity, at least some type of osseous reconstruction is required as well. If indicated, a lateral column lengthening or CC fusion may be required, but these procedures are not addressed in this article. Medial column procedures are typically performed in conjunction with a reconstruction of the diseased PTT and spring ligament, with or without a medial displacement calcaneal osteotomy (MDCO), and a lateral column procedure as discussed above. The procedures covered in this article include the Cotton osteotomy and NC fusion.

## REASONING BEHIND SURGICAL PROCEDURES THAT ADDRESS THE MEDIAL COLUMN

Flatfoot deformity includes loss of the medial arch (sagittal plane deformity), hindfoot valgus (coronal plane deformity), and forefoot abduction (axial or transverse plane deformity). This 3-dimensional deformity has been termed "dorsilateral peritalar subluxation" because abduction of the TN joint and eversion of the subtalar joint often are an integral part of the deformity. Peritalar subluxation is measured by TN coverage on an AP radiograph. Thus, the hindfoot deformity in this context can be attributed, at least in part, to the loss of stability through the medial column, as loss of the longitudinal arch through the medial column (medial column collapse) can occur through any one of the medial column joints (TN, NC or first TMT).[7]

Medial column fusion versus osteotomy is a subject of ongoing debate. Proponents of fusion cite predictable fusion rates, excellent deformity correction, and the nonessential function of the NC and TMT joints.[7–11] Advocates for the Cotton osteotomy argue that the procedure reliably restores the Meary line, obviates fusion, and is joint sparing.[5,12]

## COTTON OSTEOTOMY

The Cotton osteotomy is a dorsal opening wedge medial cuneiform osteotomy. First described in 1936 as a therapy for flatfoot to restore the tripod effect of the foot, it serves to plantar flex the first ray.[13,14]

### INDICATIONS

The Cotton osteotomy is a useful adjunct to a flatfoot reconstruction. It can help to address residual forefoot varus after correction of hindfoot valgus. Forefoot varus can be identified on physical examination. With the hindfoot reduced to neutral, the forefoot remains in a supinated position.

Consideration should also be given to using the Cotton osteotomy to address sag at the NC joint or classically with residual forefoot supination in the flexible flatfoot as well. Aiyer and colleagues[5] controlled for concomitant flatfoot procedures (eg, lateral column lengthening, tendon transfers) and showed that the Cotton osteotomy was a

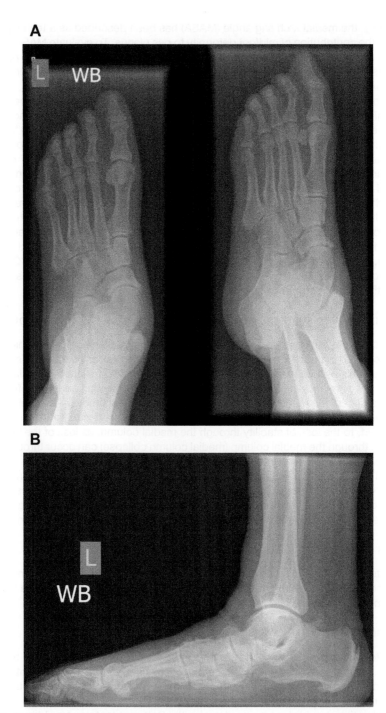

**Fig. 2.** AP (*A*) and lateral (*B*) weight-bearing radiographs of a 67-year-old man with stage III pes planus. Note the degenerative changes at the subtalar and NC joint, NC sag with dorsal joint space narrowing, and significant forefoot abduction.

useful, joint-sparing alternative to midfoot fusion when medial column stabilization was required. The Cotton procedure is also a useful adjunct to avoid additional joint fusion in cases of NC sag with severe pes planovalgus and hindfoot degenerative changes (**Figs. 2** and **3**).

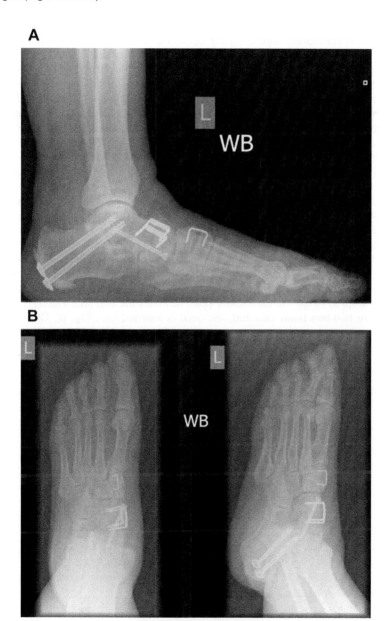

**Fig. 3.** The patient underwent medial double hindfoot fusion with gastrocnemius recession and Cotton procedure. These 3-month postoperative weight-bearing radiographs (*A, B*) show consolidating subtalar and NC fusion sites. Note significant improvement in forefoot abduction with the hindfoot fusion and improvement in NC sag with the addition of the Cotton procedure.

Contraindications to the Cotton procedure include severe degenerative changes at the NC joint and advanced deformity beyond what the typical 6- to 8-mm Cotton wedge can correct. In these circumstances, consideration for fusion is prudent.

## TECHNIQUE

The patient is positioned supine on the operating room table. A thigh tourniquet is placed and a bump under the operative hip is placed to bring the foot to neutral. If indicated, a gastrocnemius recession or Achilles lengthening is performed first. The PTT is approached next, and the appropriate procedure is completed (eg, FDL transfer to navicular, modified Kidner procedure). Before securing the final fixation medially, all osteotomies (eg, MDCO, lateral column lengthening, CC fusion) are completed and appropriate fixation is placed (**Fig. 4**). It is now critical to assess forefoot varus, and if residual varus persists, a Cotton osteotomy is indicated. The Cotton osteotomy could also be indicated based on NC sag determined preoperatively. The medial cuneiform is identified with a freer elevator using fluoroscopy (**Fig. 5**). An incision dorsal to the extensor digitorum longus (EHL) tendon is made and the EHL tendon is retracted laterally. The interval between the tibialis anterior and EHL is often used as well. A K-wire is placed in the medial cuneiform in the projected plane of the osteotomy, which is 90° perpendicular to the medial cuneiform at the central portion of the bone (see **Fig. 5**). A sagittal saw is used to create the osteotomy. It is crucial to leave the plantar cortex intact to maintain the stability of the osteotomy. Trials are then inserted from dorsal to plantar to assess correction. Typical wedge size is from 5 to 8 mm depending on the severity of the deformity. A pin distractor or laminar spreader can be helpful to hinge the osteotomy open to insert the trial (see **Fig. 7**). Once the appropriate trial has been selected, the graft is inserted (see **Fig. 8**). Graft choices

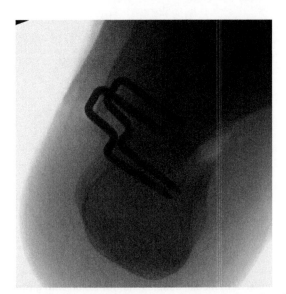

**Fig. 4.** Once the FDL tendon is harvested and provisionally transferred to the navicular, the MDCO is completed before the Cotton osteotomy is performed. Note 1-cm medial translation of tuberosity fragment. An axial view of the heel ensures that the hardware is in good position and that the tuberosity fragment is appropriately translated.

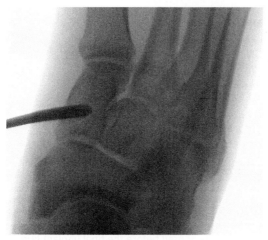

**Fig. 5.** Location of medial cuneiform with a freer elevator is helpful to place the incision for the Cotton osteotomy in the correct location.

include iliac crest autograft, allograft, or metal wedges. Dorsal fixation is used as needed depending on the press fit of the graft (**Figs. 6–9**).

After wound closure, the patient is splinted. Sutures are removed at 2 weeks, and a short-leg, non-weight-bearing cast is placed. Weight bearing in a walker boot is initiated at 6 weeks if there is evidence of radiographic healing. Shoe wear is often tolerated at 10 to 12 weeks postoperatively.

The Cotton procedure helps to restore the tripod of the foot through plantar flexion of the first ray. Several articles have shown powerful correction of Meary line, high

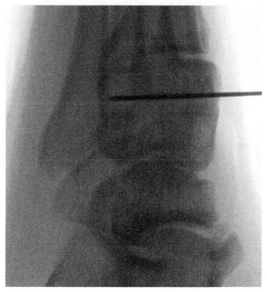

**Fig. 6.** A K-wire is placed in the medial cuneiform in the projected plane of the osteotomy, which is 90° perpendicular to the medial cuneiform at the central portion of the bone.

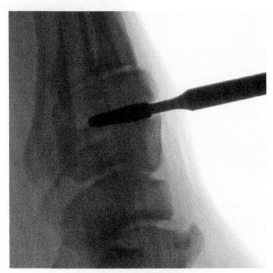

**Fig. 7.** The appropriate sized trial is used before the final implant is impacted into position. It is important to keep the plantar cortex intact to preserve the stability of the osteotomy.

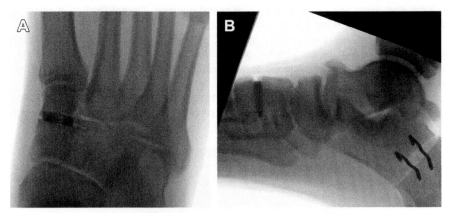

**Fig. 8.** Final construct, including Cotton osteotomy (with a metal 5-mm wedge) and MDCO with compression staples (*A*). Note the plantar cortex remains intact for the Cotton osteotomy (*B*).

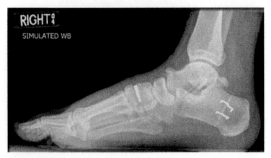

**Fig. 9.** Six-week postoperative standing radiograph showing the Cotton wedge in good position with the MDCO almost fully healed.

union rates, and excellent patient satisfaction.[5,12,15] The Cotton osteotomy is a technically straightforward procedure that should be considered in cases of NC sag without advanced NC arthrosis or residual forefoot varus after correction of hindfoot valgus (**Figs. 10–12**).

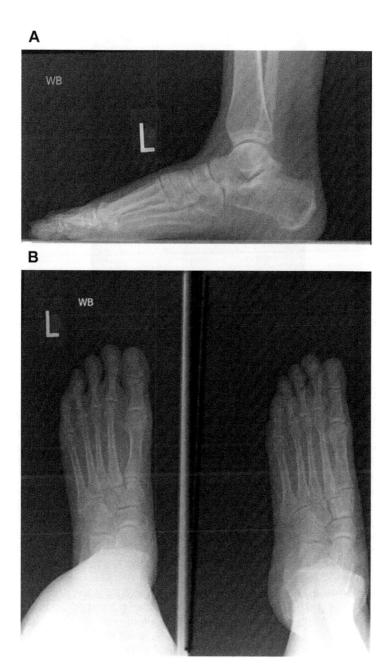

**Fig. 10.** Case example of a 51-year-old woman with PTTD and moderate pes planus. Note the NC sag on the lateral view (*A*) and uncoverage of talar head on AP view (*B*).

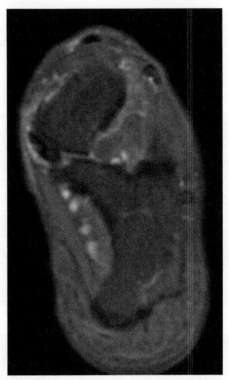

**Fig. 11.** T2 MRI of patient in **Fig. 10** showing fluid in the PTT sheath and a split tear of the tendon.

## NAVICULOCUNEIFORM FUSION

Over the years, several different procedures have been described that use NC and medial column fusion to achieve correction in flatfoot. The goal of these surgeries has been similar, to maintain hindfoot motion and improve arch height. In 1927, Miller[16] hypothesized that loss of support from the medial structures in the foot caused flatfoot deformity. He proposed NC fusion, along with first TMT fusion, achilles tendon lengthening (TAL), and PTT osteoperiosteal flap advancement as a treatment of flexible flatfoot in adolescents. Miller noted improvement in 16 patients with 2.5 years of follow-up.[2,16] In 1931, Hoke described NC fusion in both adults and adolescents. His procedure consisted of a bone block arthrodesis of the NC joint, along with PTT advancement and Achilles lengthening. In 1983, the modified Hoke-Miller procedure was described, which included NC fusion and an opening wedge osteotomy of the medial cuneiform.

In 2005, Greisberg and colleagues[7] published on medial column fusion (NC fusion, with and without TMT fusion), along with PTT debridement and FDL transfer in adult acquired flatfoot. The investigators thought that midfoot realignment and arthrodesis could improve bony relationships in some adult-acquired flatfeet with subluxation of the first TMT joint and/or sag at the medial NC joint. In 19 patients, the lateral talometatarsal angle was near normal after surgery, suggesting that a decrease in TN subluxation in the axial plane results in passive improvement in hindfoot position without

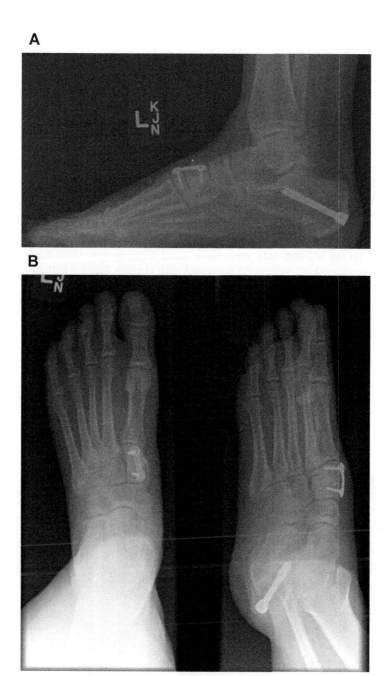

**Fig. 12.** Sixteen-month postoperative standing plain films after MDCO, FDL transfer, and Cotton osteotomy with allograft wedge and dorsal plate (*A*). Note improvement in NC sag on lateral radiograph (*B*).

direct manipulation of any hindfoot bones or joints. These observations provide evidence for a link between stability of the midfoot and alignment of the hindfoot. The investigators argued that hindfoot alignment can be improved without fusing essential joints (**Fig. 13**).

In 2013, Ajis and Geary[9] reported on 28 patients (33 feet) that underwent NC fusion for NC sag or degenerative changes at the NC joint in the context of pes planus. Ninety-seven percent of patients had a satisfactory outcome with radiographic and clinical correction of flatfoot deformity. Of note, average time to fusion was 5 months, which is longer than is seen in other foot joints.

Neglected NC arthritis can lead to progressive medial column instability. If left untreated, this can cause transfer of stress across the midfoot, including lesser metatarsal stress fractures and/or midfoot arthritis (**Figs. 14–16**).

Nonunion is the main potential complication in NC fusion. The risk is low but is worth consideration. Ford and Hamilton[17] cite up to a 7% nonunion rate in their review article. In Greisberg's seminal article on medial column stability, the nonunion rate of when both the NC and TMT joints were fused together was 15%. Barg and colleagues[10] combined NC fusion with subtalar fusion in stage II and III flatfoot deformity and had zero nonunions. Their construct had dorsal screws as well as a plantar-medial plate at the NC joint to act as a tension band. In a heavy smoker or severe diabetic, one might consider another procedure for flatfoot reconstruction given the nonunion risk associated with NC fusion.

### Technique of Naviculocuneiform Fusion

The patient is placed supine on the operating room table; a thigh tourniquet is placed, and a bump under the operative hip is placed to bring the foot to neutral. If indicated, a gastrocnemius recession if performed first. A medial approach to the foot between the medial cuneiform and the medial malleolus is then made. The incision is typically just dorsal to the PTT. The PTT is approached first and the appropriate procedure is

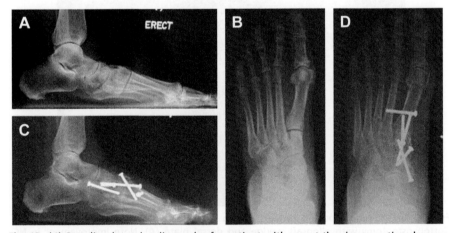

**Fig. 13.** (*A*) Standing lateral radiograph of a patient with sag at the degenerative changes and sag at the NC joint and plantar gapping at the first TMT base. (*B*) Talonavicular uncoverage noted on an AP radiograph. (*C*) Lateral radiograph 6 months after medial column arthrodesis. Note improvement in the NC sag with opening of the sinus tarsi. (*D*) AP radiograph showing significant improvement in the NC coverage. (*Courtesy of* Dr Justin Greisberg, Columbia Orthopaedics New York, NY.)

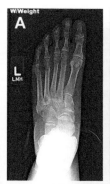
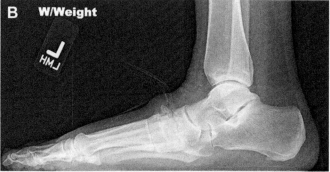

Fig. 14. AP (A) and lateral (B) weight-bearing radiographs of a 64-year-old woman with progressive midfoot pain. Note the degenerative changes apparent at the NC joint and first, second, and third TMT joints.

completed. Debridement is possible in this context, but traditional FDL transfer to the navicular is more challenging because of the NC fusion fixation. If necessary, FDL transfer to the posterior tibial stump is an option. Next, any necessary osteotomies or fusion should be completed (eg, MDCO, lateral column lengthening, CC fusion, subtalar fusion) and appropriate fixation is placed. The NC joint is then opened with a Hintermann distractor (Hintermann distractor; New-deal-Integra LifeSciences, Plainsboro, NJ, USA) using pins in the medial cuneiform and navicular. The anterior tibial tendon should be protected dorsally. One must expose all 3 NC joints for preparation. The articular cartilage is then denuded with a combination of curettes and osteotomes, and the osseous surfaces are drilled and shingled. Any necessary autograft or allograft is then placed.

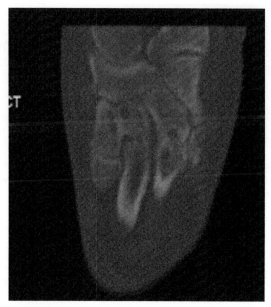

Fig. 15. Computed tomographic scan of patient in Fig. 14 showing advanced degenerative changes across the midfoot.

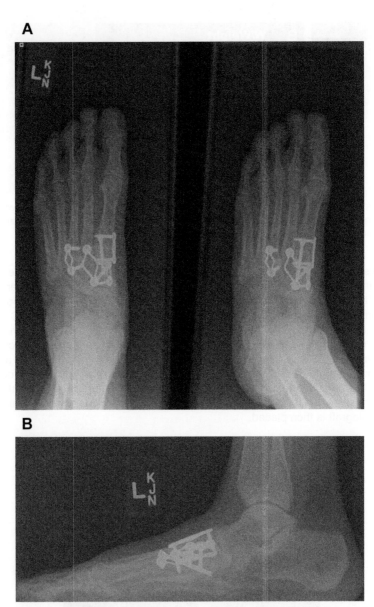

**Fig. 16.** AP (*A*) and lateral (*B*) weight-bearing radiographs 2 years after extended midfoot fusion. The patient had significant improvement in pain.

It is important to address an NC sag at this point by making an attempt to plantar flex the cuneiform bones and dorsiflex the navicular. Gentle rotation of the pin distractors in these bones can greatly help to facilitate this reduction (**Fig. 17**). With the reduction held in place, hardware is placed across the NC joint for fusion. Combinations of plates, screws, and staples have all been described (**Fig. 18**).

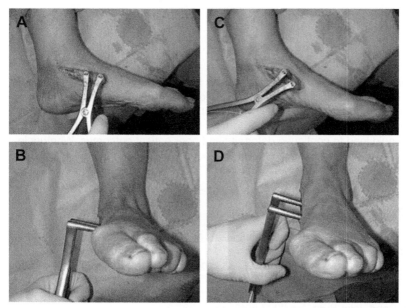

Fig. 17. (*A, B*) Pin distractor in the navicular and medial cuneiform in the uncorrected position. (*C, D*) Correction of NC sag by rotation of the pin distractor. (*From* Barg A, Brunner S, Zwicky L, et al. Subtalar and naviculocuneiform fusion for extended breakdown of the medial arch. Foot Ankle Clin 2011;16(1):75–6; with permission.)

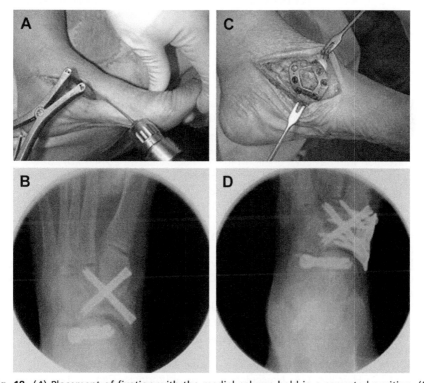

Fig. 18. (*A*) Placement of fixation with the medial column held in a corrected position. (*B*) 5.5-mm cannulated screws across NC joint. (*C, D*) Addition of medial/plantar plate for tension band effect. (*From* Barg A, Brunner S, Zwicky L, et al. Subtalar and naviculocuneiform fusion for extended breakdown of the medial arch. Foot Ankle Clin 2011;16(1):75–6; with permission.)

## SUMMARY

No single procedure is enough to address the complexity of the adult acquired flatfoot deformity. Careful physical evaluation and weight-bearing radiographs are required to form a comprehensive surgical plan. Sag at the NC joint represents an important aspect of the flatfoot deformity. Failure to address medial column instability could lead to continued deformity and poor patient outcomes. Whether in combination with other procedures or in isolation, NC fusion and Cotton osteotomy are important pieces of the armamentarium to address all aspects of the flatfoot deformity.

## REFERENCES

1. Pedowitz WJ, Kovatis P. Flatfoot in the adult. J Am Acad Orthop Surg 1995;3(5): 293–302.
2. Cohen BE, Ogden F. Medial column procedures in the acquired flatfoot deformity. Foot Ankle Clin 2007;12(2):287–99, vi.
3. Coughlin MJ, Jones CP. Hallux valgus and first ray mobility. A prospective study. J Bone Joint Surg Am 2007;89(9):1887–98.
4. Wood EV, Syed A, Geary NP. Clinical tip: the reverse coleman block test radiograph. Foot Ankle Int 2009;30(7):708–10.
5. Aiyer A, Dall GF, Shub J, et al. Radiographic correction following reconstruction of adult acquired flat foot deformity using the Cotton medial cuneiform osteotomy. Foot Ankle Int 2016;37(5):508–13.
6. Deland JT. The adult acquired flatfoot and spring ligament complex. Pathology and implications for treatment. Foot Ankle Clin 2001;6(1):129–35, vii.
7. Greisberg J, Assal M, Hansen ST Jr, et al. Isolated medial column stabilization improves alignment in adult-acquired flatfoot. Clin Orthop Relat Res 2005;(435):197–202.
8. Greisberg J, Hansen ST Jr, Sangeorzan B. Deformity and degeneration in the hindfoot and midfoot joints of the adult acquired flatfoot. Foot Ankle Int 2003; 24(7):530–4.
9. Ajis A, Geary N. Surgical technique, fusion rates, and planovalgus foot deformity correction with naviculocuneiform fusion. Foot Ankle Int 2014;35(3):232–7.
10. Barg A, Brunner S, Zwicky L, et al. Subtalar and naviculocuneiform fusion for extended breakdown of the medial arch. Foot Ankle Clin 2011;16(1):69–81.
11. Jack EA. Naviculo-cuneiform fusion in the treatment of flat foot. J Bone Joint Surg Br 1953;35-B(1):75–82.
12. Lutz M, Myerson M. Radiographic analysis of an opening wedge osteotomy of the medial cuneiform. Foot Ankle Int 2011;32(3):278–87.
13. Mosca VS. Calcaneal lengthening for valgus deformity of the hindfoot. Results in children who had severe, symptomatic flatfoot and skewfoot. J Bone Joint Surg Am 1995;77(4):500–12.
14. McCormick JJ, Johnson JE. Medial column procedures in the correction of adult acquired flatfoot deformity. Foot Ankle Clin 2012;17(2):283–98.
15. Tankson CJ. The Cotton osteotomy: indications and techniques. Foot Ankle Clin 2007;12(2):309–15, vii.
16. Miller O. A plastic flatfoot operation. J Bone Joint Surg 1927;9:84–91.
17. Ford LA, Hamilton GA. Naviculocuneiform arthrodesis. Clin Podiatr Med Surg 2004;21(1):141–56.

# Did Failure Occur Because of Medial Column Instability That Was Not Recognized, or Did It Develop After Surgery?

Anish R. Kadakia, MD*, Armen S. Kelikian, MD,
Mauricio Barbosa, MD, Milap S. Patel, DO

## KEYWORDS

- Medial column instability • Pes planovalgus • Flatfoot
- Posterior tibial tendon dysfunction

## KEY POINTS

- Medial column instability is a primary deforming force in the setting of pes planovalgus deformity.
- Consideration for medial column stabilization only after correction of the hindfoot deformity may result in creating a rigid hindfoot, compromising clinical outcomes given the secondary correction of abduction following a medial column fusion.
- Careful analysis of the lateral radiograph to determine whether the deformity is secondary to the medial column (first tarsometatarsal and/or naviculocuneiform joints) may allow superior radiographic and clinical outcomes.
- Iatrogenic creation of an excessively rigid medial column does not seem to be well tolerated and may lead to significant instability of the remaining joints in the short term and arthrosis in the long term.
- Although there is limited literature regarding the appropriate role of medial column fusion for the surgical treatment of flatfoot, it can be concluded that medial column arthrodesis should be used selectively to correct gross instability in order to maintain as much physiologic motion as possible.

## INTRODUCTION

Adult acquired flatfoot deformity (AAFD) has been addressed with an algorithmic approach based on classifications that have attempted to isolate this complex deformity into stages. Classifications allow orthopedic surgeons to discuss a pathologic

Disclosure: The authors have nothing to disclose.
Foot and Ankle Orthopedic Fellowship, Northwestern Memorial Hospital, Feinberg School of Medicine, Northwestern University, 259 East Erie, 13th Floor, Chicago, IL 60611, USA
* Corresponding author.
E-mail address: kadak259@gmail.com

entity in an academic setting; however, rigid classification systems are not able to accurately describe the nuances of a complex process and guide treatment in all cases. This statement was made by Miller[1] in 1927: "There can be no dogmatic classification of flatfoot." Although he was discussing the care of pediatric flatfoot, the concept of avoiding dogmatic treatment of this multifactorial disorder is applicable to all conditions. This difficulty is acutely noted when discussing posterior tibial tendon (PTT) dysfunction because medial column instability does not play a prominent role in the traditional classification schemes; however, it is a significant contributor to the pathologic process.

In 1989, Johnson and Strom[2] developed the first classification system (**Table 1**) for AAFD, which is based on the integrity of the PTT, hindfoot position, and flexibility of the deformity. This classification has since served as a foundation for more current classification systems. The hallmark of AAFD is attenuation of medial hindfoot supporting soft tissue structures leading to collapse of the medial longitudinal arch. Although it is a critical component of the disorder, past classifications do not emphasize medial longitudinal arch involvement or treatment options when in conjunction with AAFD.

Newer classification systems are beginning to shed some light on the medial column involvement in AAFD. In 2007, Bluman and colleagues[4] proposed a more comprehensive classification system that involved a wider spectrum of subgroups that the previous classifications did not address. These subgroups included medial column instability. The RAM (rearfoot, ankle, midfoot) Classification, described by Raikin and colleagues,[5] takes into consideration involvement of the midfoot, as well as, the hindfoot and ankle. The Grand Rapids Arch Collapse Classification, described by Anderson and colleagues,[6] describes how a myriad of problems can contribute to gastrocnemius contracture, including medial arch collapse in the later stages. Despite the detail and subclassifications that have been added to describe AAFD, each classification attempts to categorize the fluid nature of this pathologic process into defined categories. These classifications schemes serve as a guide only and cannot be relied on to dictate the appropriate treatment of each patient. On review of the treatment recommendations for medial column arthrodesis, there is no correlation with severity of the medial column deformity or whether this may substitute for hindfoot correction (**Table 2**). What is clear is that although the medial column is recognized as part of the deformity in each of classifications, the concept of the medial column as the primary deforming force is not fully understood.

The lateral first talometatarsal angle has proved to be the most discriminating radiographic parameter when evaluating patients with a flatfoot deformity.[7] Instability of the medial column is also reliably shown by analyzing the height of the medial cuneiform.[8] Although both of these measurements help to define the presence of a flatfoot deformity, neither measurement accurately defines the location of the instability, which is critical to understand in order to apply the most effective surgical correction. When evaluating lateral weight-bearing radiographs, surgeons must determine whether the medial column collapse is occurring through the talonavicular (TN), naviculocuneiform (NC), first tarsometatarsal, or a combination of joints. Failure to appropriately address the apex of the instability leads to persistent postoperative deformity. A more frustrating scenario for all parties is for all locations of instability to be addressed with excellent intraoperative correction but further medial column collapse occurs in the postoperative period, which compromises the outcome. Although this situation cannot be predicted in all situations, understanding the implications of increasing the rigidity of the hindfoot and the forefoot secondary to arthrodesis may allow surgeons to mitigate the occurrence of this

**Table 1**
**Classification system for adult acquired flatfoot deformity**

| | |
|---|---|
| Johnson & Strom (1989)[2] | Stage I |
| | Peritendinitis and/or PTT degeneration, mobile and normal hindfoot alignment, mild to moderate medial hindfoot pain, able to perform single-heel-rise test, no forefoot abduction, PTT synovitis with mild degeneration |
| | Stage 2 |
| | PTT elongation, mobile and valgus hindfoot alignment, moderate hindfoot pain over PTT, unable to perform single-heel-rise test, forefoot abduction present, marked degeneration of PTT |
| | Stage 3 |
| | PTT elongation, fixed and valgus hindfoot alignment, moderate media hindfoot pain over PTT along with lateral subfibular pain, unable to perform single-heel-rise test, forefoot abduction present, marked degeneration of PTT |
| Myerson (1996)[3]: modification of Johnson & Strom[2] classification | Stage 4 |
| | Rigid hindfoot with valgus talus angulation and lateral compartment ankle arthritis caused by deltoid attenuation |
| Bluman et al (2007)[4]: addition of subtypes to Johnson & Strom[2] and Myerson[3] classification | Stage 1A |
| | Tenderness along PTT with normal anatomy and normal radiographic findings: secondary to systemic inflammatory disease |
| | Stage 1B |
| | Tenderness along PTT with normal anatomy and normal radiographic findings |
| | Stage 1C |
| | Slight hindfoot valgus clinically and radiographically |
| | Stage 2A1 |
| | Supple hindfoot valgus, flexible forefoot varus; radiographic changes include hindfoot valgus, loss of calcanea pitch, Meary line disruption |
| | Stage 2A2 |
| | Supple hindfoot valgus, fixed forefoot varus; radiographic changes include hindfoot valgus, loss of calcanea pitch, Meary line disruption |
| | Stage 2B |
| | Same as stage 2 A2 with addition of forefoot abduction; radiographic changes include talar head uncovering and forefoot abduction |
| | Stage 2C |
| | Same as stage 2 B with addition of medial column instability, first ray dorsiflexion with hindfoot correction, sinus tarsi pain, radiographic presence of first tarsometatarsal joint plantar gapping |
| | Stage 3A |
| | Rigid hindfoot valgus, pain in sinus tarsi; radiographically there is loss of subtalar joint space, angle of Gissane sclerosis, hindfoot valgus |
| | Stage 3B |
| | Same as stage 3 A with addition of forefoot abduction |
| | Stage 4A |
| | Supple tibiotalar valgus |
| | Stage 4B |
| | Rigid tibiotalar valgus |

*(continued on next page)*

| Table 1 (*continued*) | |
|---|---|
| RAM Classification by Raikin et al (2012)[5] | Stage 1A<br>  Rearfoot: tenosynovitis of PTT<br>  Ankle: neutral alignment<br>  Midfoot: Neutral alignment<br>Stage 1B<br>  Rearfoot: PTT tendonitis without deformity<br>  Ankle: <5° valgus<br>  Midfoot: mild flexible midfoot supination<br>Stage 2A<br>  Rearfoot: flexible planovalgus (<40% talar uncoverage, <30° Meary angle, incongruence angle 20°–45°)<br>  Ankle: valgus with deltoid insufficiency (no arthritis)<br>  Midfoot: midfoot supination without radiographic instability<br>Stage 2B<br>  Rearfoot: flexible planovalgus (>40% talar uncoverage, >30° Meary angle, incongruence angle 20°–45°)<br>  Ankle: valgus with deltoid insufficiency with tibiotalar arthritis<br>  Midfoot: midfoot supination with midfoot instability and no arthritis<br>Stage 3A<br>  Rearfoot: fixed/arthritic planovalgus (<40% talar uncoverage, <30° Meary angle, incongruence angle 20°–45°)<br>  Ankle: valgus secondary to bone loss in lateral tibial plafond (deltoid normal)<br>  Midfoot: arthritis isolated to medial column (navicular–medial cuneiform or first tarsometatarsal joints)<br>Stage 3B<br>  Rearfoot: fixed/arthritic planovalgus (>40% talar uncoverage, >30° Meary angle, incongruence angle 20°–45°); not correctable through triple arthrodesis<br>  Ankle: valgus secondary to bone loss in lateral tibial plafond with deltoid normal insufficiency<br>  Midfoot: medial and middle column midfoot arthritic changes (usually with supination and/or abduction of the midfoot) |
| GRACC (2014)[6] | Type 1<br>  Affects gastrocnemius: presents with gastrocnemius equinus, plantar fasciitis, metatarsalgia, Achilles tendon pain; biomechanically there is tensile failure of posterior and plantar soft tissues<br>Type 2<br>  Affects forefoot: presents with hypermobile first ray, hallux valgus, lesser toe deformity, metatarsalgia, metatarsal stress fracture; biomechanically creating medial column incompetency with weight-bearing transfer to lesser rays<br>Type 3<br>  Affects midfoot: presents with midfoot arthritis especially at navicular–medial cuneiform, second, and third tarsometatarsal joints; biomechanically creating a transverse arch collapse<br>Type 4<br>  Affects hindfoot: presents with hindfoot valgus, peritalar subluxation, PTT disorder, lateral hindfoot/subtalar arthritis, sinus tarsi impingement; biomechanically there is medial arch collapse with spring ligament attenuation<br>Type 5<br>  Affects ankle: presents with valgus ankle arthritis; biomechanically there is deltoid ligament attenuation |

*Abbreviations:* GRACC, Grand Rapids Arch Collapse Classification; RAM, rearfoot, ankle, midfoot.

| | Table 2 | |
|---|---|---|
| **Treatment recommendations for medial column arthrodesis** | | |
| Classification | Stage with Medial Column Involvement | Surgical Treatment Addressing Medial Column Instability |
| Bluman et al (2007) [4] | Stage 2C<br>Medial column instability with radiographic presence of first TMT joint plantar gapping | Stage 2C<br>Mild instability: Cotton procedure<br>Moderate/severe instability/ arthritis: talonavicular, navicular-cuneiform, or first TMT joint arthrodesis depending on involvement |
| RAM classification (2012) | Stage 2B<br>Midfoot supination with midfoot instability and no arthritis<br>Stage 3A<br>Arthritis isolated to medial column (navicular–medial cuneiform or first tarsometatarsal joints)<br>Stage 3B<br>Medial and middle column midfoot arthritic changes (usually with supination and/or abduction of the midfoot) | Stage 2B<br>Mild instability: Cotton procedure<br>Moderate/severe instability: navicular-cuneiform or first tarsometatarsal joint arthrodesis<br>Stage 3A<br>Navicular-cuneiform or first tarsometatarsal joint arthrodesis<br>Stage 3B<br>First, second, and third TMT realignment arthrodesis in order to stabilize the medial and middle column |
| GRACC (2014) | Stage 2<br>Medial column incompetence<br>Stage 4<br>Medial arch collapse | Stage 2<br>First TMT arthrodesis<br>Stage 4<br>Flexible deformity: first TMT arthrodesis<br>Rigid deformity: talonavicular arthrodesis |

difficult complication. This article focuses on both of these aspects of medial column instability.

## MEDIAL COLUMN ARTHRODESIS FOR CORRECTION OF PES PLANOVALGUS

The primary difficulty with all reviews regarding flatfoot reconstruction is that there are no outcome scores to determine what procedures are required to improve the functional outcome. Orthopedic surgeons have focused on the improvement in radiographic angles with less attention paid to what aspects of deformity correction are associated with clinical improvement. The following discussion therefore must be approached with this critique in mind. There are 2 aspects of medial column contribution to flatfoot deformity that must be understood in order to discuss the role of surgical stabilization as an integral component of surgical reconstruction. First, the belief that the static medial restraints and stability of the medial column are components of flatfoot deformity. Many surgical algorithms place the medial column almost as an afterthought that needs to be addressed only if residual forefoot supination remains after correction of the hindfoot. However, the contribution of the medial column was initially recognized by Miller[1] in 1927. He described a surgical procedure that included an arthrodesis of the NC and first tarsometatarsal (TMT) joint, Achilles lengthening, and tightening of an osteoperiosteal flap of the medial navicular/cuneiform/first metatarsal without addressing the hindfoot. At 2.5 years of follow-up, no loss of the medial arch correction was noted; however, there is no radiographic analysis given in the article. Hoke[9] presented the first published

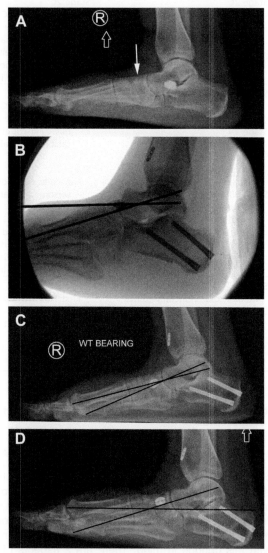

**Fig. 1.** Preoperative lateral radiograph (*A*) of a patient who failed a prior sinus tarsi implant procedure and who presented with persistent symptomatic complaints with evidence of NC collapse (*white arrow*). Intraoperative correction (*B*) was performed with a medial slide calcaneal osteotomy (medial displacement calcaneal osteotomy [MDCO]), FDL tendon transfer, gastrocnemius recession, and allograft spring ligament reconstruction. Correction was thought to be appropriate with elevation of the talar head. Three-month postoperative (*C*) radiographs note mild loss of correction through the NC joint. However, at 6 months (*D*), note the increasing loss of correction through failure of the NC joint. In hindsight, an isolated NC fusion may have been more appropriate in this patient as opposed to a spring ligament reconstruction.

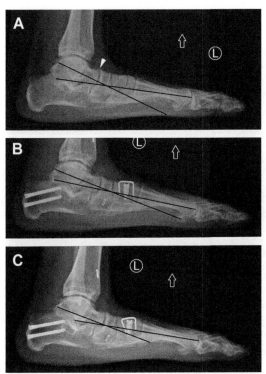

**Fig. 2.** Preoperative lateral radiograph (*A*) with deformity centered at the level of the NC joint. Note the lack of subluxation of the talonavicular (TN) joint (*white arrowhead*). Three months postoperative (*B*), mild improvement in the deformity is noted following an MDCO, FDL tendon transfer, spring ligament reconstruction, gastrocnemius recession, and Cotton osteotomy. However, near-complete recurrence of the deformity is noted (*C*) 6 months postoperatively secondary to continued collapse through the NC joint.

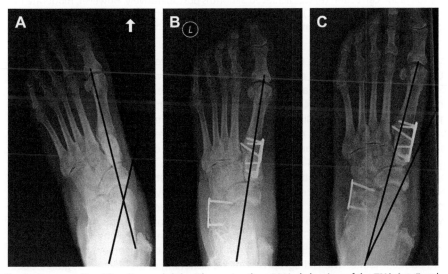

**Fig. 3.** Preoperative AP radiograph (*A*) with greater than 50% abduction of the TN joint. Excellent coronal plane correction (*B*) was thought to be achieved at 3 months following an MDCO, lateral collateral ligament (LCL), first TMT arthrodesis, spring ligament reconstruction, and FDL tendon transfer. However, at 1 year (*C*), despite bony union, loss of correction occurred, which was thought to be secondary to a failure to address the NC instability (**Fig. 4**).

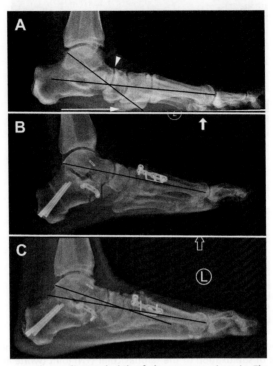

**Fig. 4.** Lateral preoperative radiograph (*A*) of the same patient in **Fig. 3**, with complete collapse of the medial column with contact of the cuneiform with the floor (*white arrow*). Note the lack of dorsal subluxation of the navicular relative to the talus (*white arrowhead*). This finding should alert the surgeon to the presence of medial column instability. Excellent sagittal plane correction (*B*) was achieved 3 months postoperatively. However, moderate loss of correction was noted at (*C*) 1 year secondary to persistent instability of the NC joint with associated loss of coronal plane correction (see **Fig. 3**).

case of the use of an NC fusion to treat AAFD. His technique used a bone block fusion of the NC joint and open Achilles lengthening, with the use of postoperative casting without internal fixation. Although limited in the data that were presented in the article, because only 4 cases (3 pediatric and 1 adult) were presented, radiographs (all 4 cases) and clinical photographs (3 pediatric) were presented showing correction of the sagittal deformity. However, this reliance on a single point of correction for a multiplanar deformity in adolescents did not withstand the test of time. Seymour[10] reviewed 32 feet in 17 patients who underwent an NC fusion for correction of a flexible flatfoot at 16 to 19 years postoperative. He evaluated the same population as was reviewed by Jack[11] (operative surgeon in all cases) at a follow-up of 15 months to 5 years postoperative. Although initial results by Jack[11] were noted to be good to excellent in 82% of patients, this deteriorated to 50% at the final follow-up by Seymour.[10] The 16 feet deemed unsatisfactory by Seymour[10] all had pain that limited activity with restriction of movement at the midtarsal and subtalar joints. The radiographs showed flattening of arch with a negative declination of the talus. Most noteworthy, all of these patients noted arthritic changes in the TN and subtalar joints. However, the review by Seymour[10] is the only article that reviews the long-term complications of an NC arthrodesis. Multiple causal factors may contribute to the hindfoot arthrosis: adjacent joint stress, failure to correct the hindfoot (calcaneal osteotomy), and/or failure relieve dynamic stress (gastrocne- mius recession or Achilles lengthening). His data should serve as a warning for readers if the decision is made to proceed with aggressive medial column fusion as a routine part of a treatment algorithm.

In addition, there is evidence that the medial column stabilization not only corrects the sagittal plane deformity but also secondarily corrects the coronal plane defor- mity. Greisberg and colleagues[12] showed a mean improvement in the anteroposte- rior (AP) TN coverage of 14° (range 1°–30°) in 19 patients who underwent medial column fusion (first TMT, NC, combined first TMT and NC) with associated augmen- tation of the PTT and gastrocnemius recession in most patients. The follow-up period was a maximum of 6 months, making it difficult to determine the long-term durability of the correction and risk of adjacent joint disease in their patient popula- tion. Ajis and Geary[13] reviewed a series of 20 skeletally mature patients who under- went an NC fusion for pes planovalgus deformity. Of these patients, 8 had a Cobb split anterior tibial tendon transfer, 2 underwent a medial displacement calcaneal osteotomy, and 7 patients had gastrocnemius recessions. Importantly, no patient underwent a lateral column lengthening. Follow-up was noted to be short term

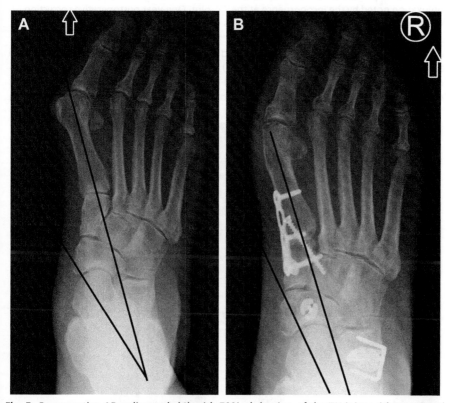

**Fig. 5.** Preoperative AP radiograph (*A*) with 50% abduction of the TN joint with associated hallux valgus deformity. Improvement in the coronal plane deformity was noted at 1 year postoperative (*B*) following an MDCO, LCL, gastrocnemius recession, spring ligament recon- struction, and Lapidus. Critically, insufficient correction of the hallux deformity is noted, with approximately 20% abduction of the TN joint. The patient is clinically satisfied despite failure to completely correct the abduction.

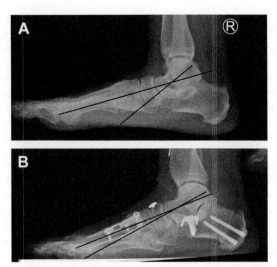

**Fig. 6.** Lateral preoperative radiograph (*A*) of the patient in **Fig. 5** with clear evidence of TN subluxation noted by the incongruence at the TN joint. One-year postoperative correction (*B*) was excellent and maintained because all sites of instability were appropriately addressed.

and patients were followed until they noted clinical and radiographic union, with the longest duration of healing noted to be 60.3 weeks (mean, 21.7 weeks). Investigators noted an improvement of the lateral talo–first metatarsal angle from −12.3° to −5.2°, with concomitant improvement of the AP talo-first metatarsal angle from

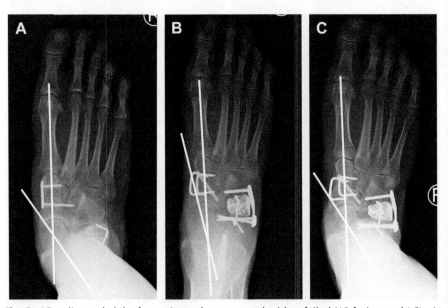

**Fig. 7.** AP radiograph (*A*) of a patient who presented with a failed NC fusion and LCL. At 3 months (*B*), excellent correction was thought to be achieved following a revision NC fusion, LCL (calcaneocuboid (CC) fusion was required because of prior joint violation), MDCO, FDL transfer, and gastrocnemius recession. However, at 1 year, near-complete recurrence of the deformity (*C*) was noted with collapse through the TN joint.

14.1° to 7.4°. The use of rigid internal fixation along with preparation of all 3 facets of the NC joint was associated with a 97% rate of arthrodesis. The significant limitation in this study is the lack of long-term follow-up and functional outcomes. However, the ability of an isolated medial column fusion to correct both sagittal and coronal plane parameters without the need for a lateral column lengthening has been clearly shown. More credence was given to the concept of medial column instability as a more relevant contributor to flatfoot deformity by Kang and colleagues,[14] whose team showed that the lateral column is not significantly shorter in patients with

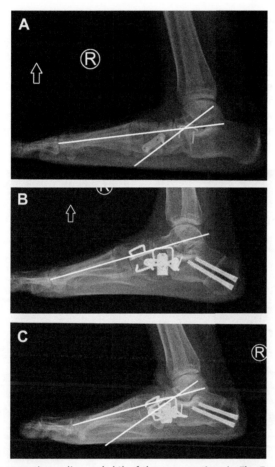

**Fig. 8.** Lateral preoperative radiograph (*A*) of the same patient in **Fig. 7** with clear collapse of the NC joint with a negative talar declination angle. At 3 months postoperative (*B*), complete restoration of sagittal balance was thought to be achieved. Radiographic collapse (*C*) is noted at 1 year with failure through the TN joint because there was union of the both the NC and CC lengthening arthrodesis based on computed tomography (CT) scan. On reexamination of the patient, the right foot was similar in appearance to the left asymptomatic foot, with complete patient satisfaction because she was able to return to all prior activities without pain. This case exemplifies that the goal of surgery is to restore patients to their preinjury/predeformity states, as opposed to theoretic radiographic parameters. Others may argue that this case is a prime example of the saying, "Better lucky than good."

AAFD compared with normal patients. Although lengthening the lateral column can reliably correct the abduction deformity, Deland and colleagues[15] showed that correction of the abduction to adduction (defined as a lateral incongruence angle >5°, a talar uncoverage angle >8°, and a talo-first metatarsal angle >8°) produced worse functional outcomes than slight undercorrection. These findings have led the authors to pursue correction of the abduction through what is thought to be a more physiologic correction by addressing the medial column instability as opposed to routine lateral column lengthening in patients who have less than 50% abduction.

## FAILURE TO ADDRESS MEDIAL COLUMN INSTABILITY

Routine use of a medial displacement calcaneal osteotomy and flexor digitorum longus (FDL) tendon transfer is likely insufficient to achieve radiographic correction of most patients with symptomatic flatfoot deformity. Identification of medial column instability on a weight-bearing lateral radiograph is not difficult and allows the surgeon to determine which additional procedures may be required to correct the radiographic deformity. The use of a lateral radiograph with the patient performing a reverse Coleman block test as described by Ajis and Geary[13] may improve the

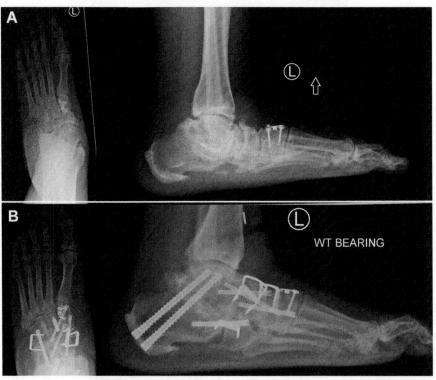

**Fig. 9.** Preoperative AP and lateral (A) radiographs of a patient who presented for revision correction of his AAFD with clear arthritic changes and collapse of the triple joint complex and NC joint. Successful correction of the deformity was achieved at 1 year (B); however, this construct may lead to instability of the first TMT joint or the deltoid ligament secondary the rigidity of the construct.

ability to identify medial column instability. Close inspection of postoperative radiographs shows the subtle changes that occur when the medial column is not addressed. Progressive loss of correction is inevitable, compromising the radiographic parameters; however, again the clinical relevance of subtle loss of correction has yet to be determined (**Fig. 1**). The use of a Cotton osteotomy to plantarflex the medial column has a reliable union rate and has shown clinical and radiographic improvement in sagittal radiographic parameters.[16] In the presence of NC instability, despite what is thought to be excellent intraoperative correction

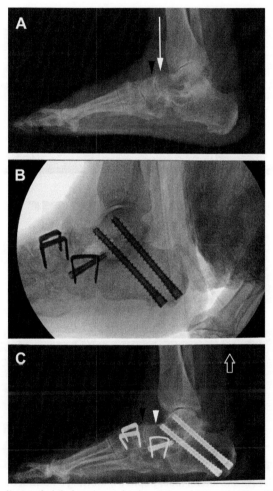

**Fig. 10.** Lateral radiograph (*A*) showing subtalar, CC, and NC arthritis with mild collapse of the medial column at the NC joint. Note the position of the talus (*white arrow*) relative to the navicular (*black arrowhead*) with no evidence of peritalar subluxation. Intraoperative fluoroscopy (*B*) of a combined subtalar, CC, and NC fusion was thought to achieve appropriate correction without resultant deformity or collapse of the TN joint. Note the change at 1 year in the position of the TN joint (*C*) with a clear alteration of the relationship of the navicular (*black arrowhead*) relative to the now more plantar talus (*white arrowhead*). The rigidity that was created within the NC joint was compensated by reciprocal instability of the TN joint in the postoperative period.

from the osteotomy, recurrence of deformity and disappointment in the clinical appearance occurs in the setting of untreated NC instability (**Fig. 2**). Although the Cotton osteotomy is simple and can be effective, it cannot substitute for stabilization of the NC or first TMT joint. In many cases, the use of a first TMT arthrodesis has been advocated as a way to improve medial column instability and plantarflex the medial column. However, using the first TMT as a proxy for NC instability does not achieve a long-term solution (**Figs. 3** and **4**). However, the presence of hallux valgus in conjunction with a pes planovalgus deformity should attune the surgeon

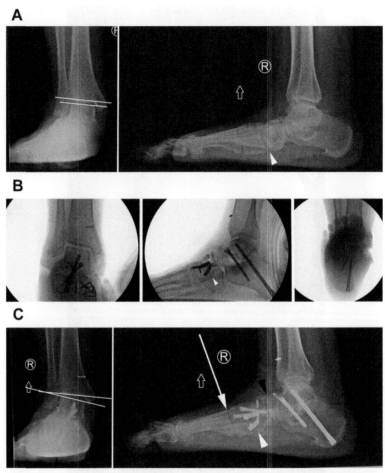

**Fig. 11.** Preoperative AP and lateral radiographs (A) showing a flatfoot deformity with clear collapse at the NC joint with a neutral tibiotalar joint. Intraoperative fluoroscopy (B) was performed secondary to the instability of the subtalar joint and obesity with associated NC fusion and allograft spring ligament reconstruction. Appropriate alignment was thought to be achieved with correction of the sagittal plane deformity and restoration of a neutral axis of the hindfoot. Medial column failure occurred in this case through the deltoid ligament with subsequent ankle valgus (C). The remaining medial column, including the first TMT joint (*white arrow*), NC arthrodesis (*white arrowhead*), and TN joint (*black arrowhead*) maintained their positions, which may explain why the collapse occurred through the deltoid ligament.

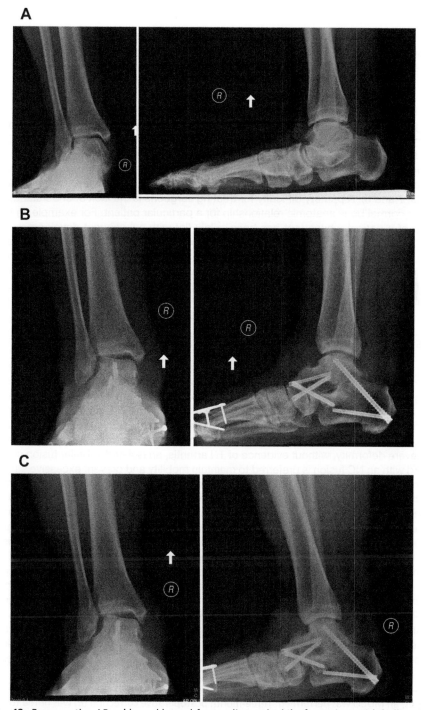

**Fig. 12.** Preoperative AP ankle and lateral foot radiographs (*A*) of a patient with hallux rigidus combined with a symptomatic severe pes planus deformity. Note the mild ankle valgus on the AP radiograph. Because of the severe hindfoot instability and early arthritic changes noted on CT scan, a triple arthrodesis, first metatarsophalangeal (MTP) arthrodesis, with an Achilles lengthening was performed. In addition, in an attempt to minimize the risk of ankle

to the presence of first TMT instability. In this setting, a first TMT arthrodesis is the appropriate procedure to correct both the coronal and sagittal plane deformity. When reviewing the radiographs, plantarflexion of the talar head relative to the navicular (true dorsolateral peritalar subluxation) denotes that the instability is occurring through the TN joint and not the NC joint. In these situations, addressing the hindfoot disorder primarily (spring ligament reconstruction and/or lateral column lengthening) is more appropriate than adding an NC fusion (**Figs. 5** and **6**). The primary concern for surgeons is how to maintain correction without creating excessive hindfoot rigidity through the use of overlengthening of the lateral column or subtalar arthrodesis. In many cases, despite addressing all observed components of the deformity, correction is not maintained but the patient is completely satisfied (**Figs. 7** and **8**). A primary difficulty for treating surgeons is the lack of understanding of the normal bony anatomic relationship for a particular patient. For example, in the case of a patient whose foot has been mildly flat with subsequent development of posterior tibial tendon dysfunction and worsening collapse, attempting to correct the foot to an idealistic neutral may result in an inappropriately stiff foot or force the stresses to collapse another aspect of the medial column. However, clinicians do not have a complete understanding of the primary pathologic process in flatfoot deformity, as is made clear by the controversies addressed in this publication and the difficulty in creating an accurate biomechanical model.

## POSTRECONSTRUCTION MEDIAL COLUMN INSTABILITY

The increased stress imparted on adjacent joints following a triple arthrodesis with subsequent degenerative changes has been well documented.[8–11,17] Barg and colleagues[17] noted that extension of a triple arthrodesis to include the NC joint stiffens the posterior aspect of the medial arch, overloading the distal joints and resulting in medial column collapse. However, in some situations, this cannot be avoided if both joints are clinically symptomatic (**Fig. 9**). They therefore recommend that in cases of severe deformity, without evidence of TN arthritis, an isolated subtalar fusion combined with an NC fusion is preferred to maintain mobility and prevent excessive stress to the remaining joints. The authors have used this concept in our practice; however, we have noted that there is a tendency for the medial column to collapse at the TN joint in the postoperative period (**Fig. 10**). Although this collapse does not seem to compromise function in the small subset of patients who have undergone this procedure, absolute rigidity of the medial column may not be biomechanically appropriate because the foot shows instability through the adjacent joints in the postoperative period in some cases. More critically, and even more difficult to address, is instability through the deltoid ligament (**Fig. 11A–C**). This serious complication may only be avoidable by minimizing the creation of rigidity in the hindfoot and accepting a compromised radiographic correction of the flatfoot deformity.

   Although not previously described, the authors have noted that, in patients who have a pes planovalgus deformity in addition to hallux rigidus, arthrodesis of the hallux in conjunction with a hindfoot fusion may result in a significant increase in stress

---

valgus, an MDCO was performed. Three-month postoperative correction (*B*) was noted to be satisfactory with improvement in the alignment of the first TMT and NC joints. However, the ankle valgus was noted to worsen. At 1 year postoperative (*C*), severe collapse of the NC and first TMT joint was noted with additional worsening of the ankle valgus. The added stiffness imparted from a first MTP arthrodesis was thought to contribute to failure of the residual medial column.

across the medial column, resulting in rapid loss of correction. This concept is akin to what was described by Barg and colleagues,[17] who noted that creating an extended hindfoot fusion results in rapid collapse of the first TMT joint and loss of correction. When the authors encounter this scenario, we now choose to use joint-sparing surgery for the hallux in all cases to minimize this risk (**Fig. 12**A–C).

## SUMMARY

Medial column instability is a primary deforming force in the setting of pes planovalgus deformity. Consideration for medial column stabilization only after correction of the hindfoot deformity may result in creating a rigid hindfoot, compromising clinical outcomes given the secondary correction of abduction following a medial column fusion. Careful analysis of the lateral radiograph to determine whether the deformity is secondary to the medial column (first TMT and/or NC joints), which is best served by a medial column arthrodesis, or true peritalar subluxation that may be superiorly treated with hindfoot stabilization (lateral collateral ligament or spring ligament reconstruction) may allow superior radiographic and clinical outcomes. Iatrogenic creation of an excessively rigid medial column does not seem to be well tolerated and may lead to significant instability of the remaining joints in the short term and arthrosis in the long term. Despite clear evidence that a medial column arthrodesis is effective in correcting the radiographic parameters of a flatfoot deformity, this correction has not been evaluated for long-term clinical outcomes since 1967, when a deterioration of function and increase in pain over time was shown. Although there is limited literature regarding the appropriate role of medial column fusion for the surgical treatment of flatfoot, it can be concluded with some confidence that medial column arthrodesis should be used selectively to correct gross instability in order to maintain as much physiologic motion as possible.

## REFERENCES

1. Miller OL. A plastic flat foot operation. JBJS 1927;9(1):84–91.
2. Johnson KA, Strom DE. Tibialis posterior tendon dysfunction. Clin Orthop Relat Res 1989;239:196–206.
3. Myerson MS. Adult acquired flatfoot deformity: treatment of dysfunction of the posterior tibial tendon. JBJS Am 1996;78:780–92.
4. Bluman EM, Title CI, Myerson MS. Posterior tibial tendon rupture: a refined classification system. Foot Ankle Clin 2007;12:233–49.
5. Raikin SM, Winters BS, Daniel JN. The RAM Classification: a novel approach to adult acquired flatfoot. Foot Ankle Clin 2012;17:169–81.
6. Anderson JG, Donald BR, Erik EB, et al. Gastrocnemius recession. Foot Ankle Clin 2014;19(4):767–86.
7. Younger AS, Sawatzky B, Dryden P. Radiographic assessment of adult flatfoot. Foot Ankle Int 2005;26(10):820–5.
8. Arangio GA, Wasser T, Rogman A. Radiographic comparison of standing medial cuneiform arch height in adults with and without acquired flatfoot deformity. Foot Ankle Int 2006;27(8):636–8.
9. Hoke M. An operation for the correction of extremely relaxed flat feet. JBJS Am 1931;13:773–83.
10. Seymour N. The late results of naviculo-cuneiform fusion. J Bone Joint Surg Br 1967;49(3):558–9.
11. Jack EA. Naviculo-cuneiform fusion in the treatment of flat foot. J Bone Joint Surg Br 1953;35(1):75–82.

12. Greisberg J, Assal M, Hansen ST Jr, et al. Isolated medial column stabilization improves alignment in adult-acquired flatfoot. Clin Orthop Relat Res 2005;435: 197–202.
13. Ajis A, Geary N. Surgical technique, fusion rates, and planovalgus foot deformity correction with naviculocuneiform fusion. Foot Ankle Int 2014;35(3):232–7.
14. Kang S, Charlton TP, Thordarson DB. Lateral column length in adult flatfoot deformity. Foot Ankle Int 2013;34:392–7.
15. Deland JT, Otis JC, Lee KT, et al. Lateral column lengthening with calcaneocuboid fusion: range of motion in the triple joint complex. Foot Ankle Int 1995;16: 729–33.
16. Tankson CJ. The cotton osteotomy: indications and techniques. Foot Ankle Clin 2007;12(2):309–15.
17. Barg A, Brunner S, Zwicky L, et al. Subtalar and naviculocuneiform fusion for extended breakdown of the medial arch. Foot Ankle Clin 2011;16(1):69–81.

# Calcaneal Osteotomies
## Pearls and Pitfalls

Stephen Greenfield, MD*, Bruce Cohen, MD

## KEYWORDS

- Calcaneal osteotomy • Heel slide • Hindfoot valgus

## KEY POINTS

- The medializing calcaneal osteotomy (MDCO) is a highly useful and efficient tool that should be considered in the algorithm of surgical correction for adult acquired flatfoot deformity.
- When radiographic and clinical examination determines hindfoot valgus to be a component of the existing deformity, the MDCO has clear benefits.
- A simple oblique incision with minimal surgical risk is used for the approach.
- The osteotomy is easy to perform and has a reliable impact on hindfoot valgus, allowing in-depth preoperative planning.

## INTRODUCTION: NATURE OF THE PROBLEM

Adult acquired flatfoot deformity is the cumulative result of multiple linked pathologic conditions. An unfavorable bony structure, or pes planus, causes excess load on the medial soft tissues. Repetitive loading results in posterior tibial tendon overload and subsequent failure, as well as attenuation of the spring ligament. This, in turn, allows for further collapse and failure of the bony arch resulting in increased forefoot abduction and peritalar subluxation and hindfoot valgus.[1] This article focuses on correction of hindfoot valgus through the use of the medializing calcaneal osteotomy (MDCO).

## INDICATIONS OR CONTRAINDICATIONS
### Indications

- Stage II flatfoot with hindfoot valgus
- Residual valgus deformity after prior subtalar fusion

An algorithmic approach is critical for the treatment of flatfoot deformity. Joint-sparing procedures are performed for flexible deformities and a sequential approach is used to determine the procedures used. Each procedure aims to correct a specific

The authors have nothing to disclose.
OrthoCarolina Foot & Ankle Institute, 2001 Vail Avenue, Suite 200B, Charlotte, NC 28207, USA
* Corresponding author.
*E-mail address:* stephen.greenfield@orthocarolina.com

component. MDCO should be considered with hindfoot valgus as both an effective way to correct valgus deformity but also mitigate the contribution of Achilles loading to deformity progression. Nyska and colleagues[2] demonstrated in a cadaveric model of flatfoot deformity that Achilles loading, in the setting of valgus deformity, exacerbated the flatfoot deformity. Following MDCO, Achilles loading contributed less to arch collapse, allowing them to conclude that MDCO serves to correct existing deformity while altering the natural history of flatfoot deformity.

### Contraindications

- Isolated forefoot deformity
- Subtalar arthritis and limited motion

Multiple studies have studied changes in radiographic parameters as a function of MDCO.[3,4] Consistently, the MDCO has been shown to not effectively correct forefoot abduction or peritalar subluxation. Therefore, patients with primarily forefoot abduction are best treated with osteotomies aimed at correcting this deformity. Likewise, in the presence of subtalar arthritis with a rigid subtalar joint, the authors recommend a limited fusion approach.

## SURGICAL TECHNIQUE OR PROCEDURE
### Preoperative Planning

Preoperative planning should include detailed radiographic assessment of hindfoot valgus. Two views are commonly referenced in the literature, the hindfoot alignment view, and the long axial view. Depending on how the deformity is measured, there are differences in interobserver and intraobserver reliabilities.[5,6] The authors' preferred method of quantification of hindfoot deformity is the magnitude of the moment arm as defined by the perpendicular distance from the extended tibial axis to the weightbearing apex of the calcaneus, as described in multiple studies.[5,7,8] Alternatively, the angular deformity, defined by the angle between the tibial axis and long axis of the calcaneus, can be used.[6] Ellis and colleagues[8] demonstrated a linear relationship between magnitude of intraoperative shift and the change in the moment arm, as measured on the hindfoot alignment view. Thus, a recommended intraoperative shift can be calculated from preoperative imaging. The clinical implications regarding accuracy of correction when using this approach has yet to be studied.

### Preparation and patient positioning

- The patient is positioned supine with an ipsilateral bump placed at the hip. For medial procedures, this bump can be removed to improve exposure.
- A thigh tourniquet is placed. An ankle tourniquet is contraindicated given the need for Achilles mobility.

### Surgical approach

- A standard oblique lateral approach to the calcaneus is made. The skin incision should extend from just anterior to the Achilles insertion at the superior calcaneal tuber to the plantar soft spot near the origin of the plantar fascia (**Fig. 1**A). This is posterior to the peroneal sheath.
- For alternative osteotomy techniques, a less oblique incision can be used.
- The sural nerve is not typically directly visualized in this approach but care still should be taken to avoid damage or traction injury.
- Once protected, the exposure is deepened down to periosteum (see **Fig. 1**B).

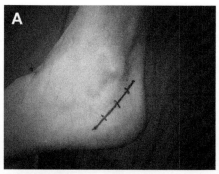 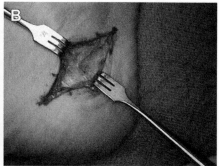

**Fig. 1.** (A) Oblique lateral incision is made posterior to the peroneal tendons. (B) Careful dissection to periosteum, protecting sural nerve.

## Osteotomy Technique

- Hohmann retractors are inserted above the calcaneal tuberosity just anterior to the Achilles and below calcaneal tuber. Standard retractors can maintain adequate central exposure (**Fig. 2**A).
- The osteotomy trajectory is marked with electrocautery (see **Fig. 2**B). Alternatively, small K-wires can be used and lateral fluoroscopic imaging obtained.
- A narrow fan-blade microsagittal saw is used to cut from lateral to medial with the Hohmann retractors protecting posterior and inferior soft tissues. Common mistakes include overpenetration and overheating of bone. Narrow osteotomes can be used to compete the osteotomy and irrigation should be used to prevent overheating at the saw-bone interface (see **Fig. 2**C).
- A combination of osteotomy and smooth lamina spreaders are used to distract at the osteotomy site and elongate surrounding soft tissues. This allows adequate mobilization of the heel fragment.
- A freer elevator is used to verify the anterior calcaneus edge is smooth (because this will inhibit translation) and soft tissues are loose (see **Fig. 2**D).
- Shift according to preoperative plan. Care should be taken to dorsiflex the ankle as the heel is shifted to lock in the translation.
- Insert a K-wire for temporary fixation. Useful landmarks include the glabrous skin junction at the central heel. The K-wire should aim laterally (to compensate for the medial shift) and toward the level of the talar head (goal is perpendicular to osteotomy) (see **Fig. 2**E)
- Check lateral and axial radiograph to verify alignment. In addition to medialization, we try and prevent shortening of the Achilles by slight plantar displacement of the tuber (see **Fig. 2**F, G).
- Final fixation can be achieved with a variety of techniques. Lateral based plate and staple constructs are available but our preference is a single, large, percutaneous cannulated screw (see **Fig. 2**H).
  - Goal should be compression perpendicular to the osteotomy site. Partially threaded versus variable compression screws are recommended.
- Smooth lateral step-off is performed with a rasp versus a rongeur.
- Closure is completed with subcutaneous and skin closure of choice.

## Alternative Osteotomy Technique

A step-cut osteotomy can also be performed. This osteotomy is an extra-articular osteotomy as well, which allows both medial displacement and lengthening of the

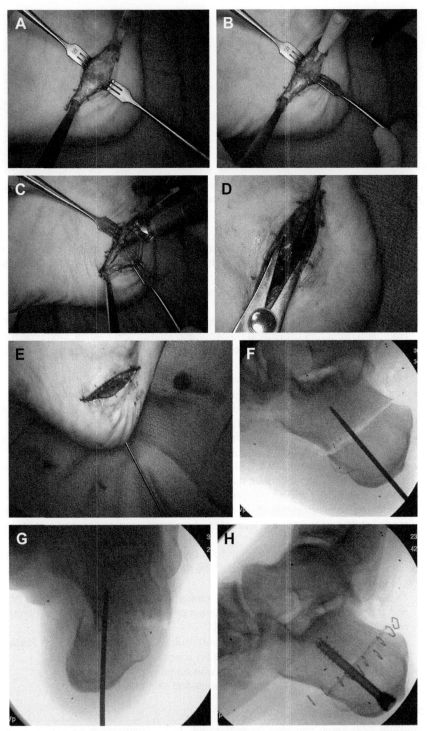

**Fig. 2.** (*A*) Retractors placed above and below calcaneus at apices of incision. (*B*) Electrocautery is used to delineate osteotomy trajectory. (*C*) Sagittal saw is used for osteotomy. Take

calcaneus. This differs from the distal step-cut osteotomy because this is posterior in the tuberosity and extra-articular in nature.

- Same skin incision is used but is lengthened both proximally and distally.
- The sural nerve will likely be encountered in this more extensile incision and should be protected. Likewise, the peroneal tendons are elevated dorsally at the level of the peroneal tubercle and protected throughout the case.
- A long step-cut osteotomy is performed with the posterior vertical limb beginning at the superior calcaneus. The long horizontal limb extends to approximately the peroneal tubercle (**Fig. 3**A). The distal vertical limb extends plantarly.
- The osteotomy is competed with microsagittal saw and osteotome. The tuberosity is shifted medially and can be rotated to lengthen the calcaneus with a pin-based distractor.
- The lengthened regions are held in the lengthened position with allograft or autograft wedges, or commercially available metal wedges (see **Fig. 3**B).
- The construct can be stabilized with various screw constructs.

This is an attractive option for several reasons. The distraction feature imparts excellent stability on the osteotomy while the large horizontal limb provides theoretic benefit in terms of successful union. This osteotomy has some early reports of excellent deformity correction and absence of progression or occurrence of arthrosis of the calcaneocuboid joint.[9]

## COMPLICATIONS AND MANAGEMENT

As with all osteotomies, the calcaneal osteotomy has multiples associated risks:

- Injury to the sural nerve
- Injury to medial structures (tibial nerve or artery)
- Nonunion or malunion with loss of correction.

Neurovascular injury is a reported complication associated with the posterior calcaneal osteotomy. Most commonly, the oblique incision can place the sural nerve or its branches at risk. Care should be taken when dissecting in subcutaneous tissue. However, once the sural nerve is protected, there are no at-risk lateral structures. There are reports of medial neurovascular injury. Cadaveric dissections were studied to assess proximity of the oblique osteotomy to medial structures.[10] Osteotomies were made in standard fashion followed by medial dissections to assess proximity of each neurovascular structure to the osteotomy. On average, 4 neurovascular structures crossed the osteotomy site. Most often, these were branches of either the lateral plantar nerve (LPN) or the posterior tibial artery (PTA). Rarely, the LPN, or the PTA itself, crossed the site. The medial plantar nerve and its branches were never at risk. Given the variability in location and number of structures, the authors recommend caution when completing the osteotomy to avoid medial neurovascular injury.

---

care to avoid overpenetration. Osteotomes are useful to complete osteotomy. (*D*) Lamina spreader (smooth) is used to displace osteotomy, relax tissues. Freer elevator is used to mobilize medial tissue and assess cut. (*E*) Manual shift of tuber with provisional K-wire fixation. (*F*) Lateral image demonstrating osteotomy after medial shift and slight plantar advancement. (*G*) Axial image demonstrating significant medial translation. (*H*) Lateral image postfixation with partially threaded compression screw.

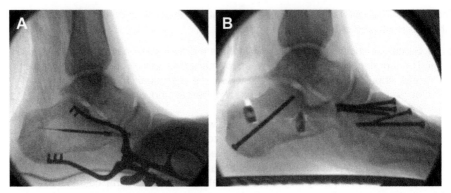

**Fig. 3.** (*A*) Lateral image demonstrating horizontal component of Z-type osteotomy. (*B*) Z-type osteotomy postfixation.

Nonunion or malunion are rare complications associated with this osteotomy. In our experience, this has been limited to patients with systemic comorbidities, often in the form of pathologic vitamin D deficiency. One patient required repeat revision fusion for a nonunion. In addition to the necessary medical treatment, revision surgery included increased fixation with biologic supplementation in the form of osteoinductive modalities and ultimately autologous bone graft (**Fig. 4**). Despite the large cancellous interface, the authors recommend avoiding prolonged saw use and subsequent thermal necrosis of the bone as a way to minimize the risk of nonunion.

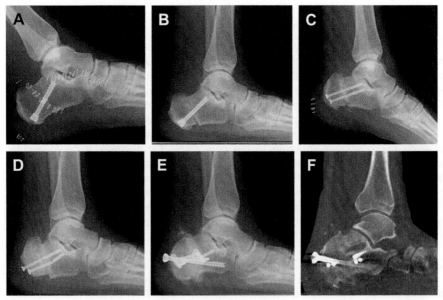

**Fig. 4.** (*A*) Lateral image of postoperative MDCO. (*B*) Loss of fixation with evidence of nonunion. (*C*) Revision fusion with multiple points of fixation and osteoinductive adjuvant treatment. (*D*) Persistent nonunion and hardware failure. (*E*) Revision MDCO with autogenous bone grafting. (*F*) Computed tomography scan demonstrating fusion.

## POSTOPERATIVE CARE

Calcaneal osteotomies require protected weightbearing until bony union. Typically, this procedure is performed in conjunction with multiple other procedures with similar postoperative requirements, thus not imposing additional limitations on activity:

- The patient is placed in postoperative splint and instructed to not bear weight on the operative leg.
- The patient is transitioned to cast versus boot at 2 weeks; continued nonweightbearing.
- Range of motion allowed at 4 weeks if in boot.
- Begin weightbearing at 4 to 6 weeks in boot if lateral radiograph confirms maintenance of position and fixation. Clinical discomfort at the osteotomy site warrants further investigation and possible prolonged nonweightbearing.
- The boot is typically discontinued at 10 to 12 weeks with radiographic confirmation of adequate healing and correction of deformity.

## OUTCOMES

The medial displacing calcaneal osteotomy is the workhorse surgical procedure for correction of hindfoot valgus. Research has shown the osteotomy to affect radiographic alignment, pressure distributions in the foot and ankle, and patient-reported pain and function.

### Radiographic Correction

Long-term outcomes of MDCO with flexor digitorum longus (FDL) tendon transfer are generally favorable. Like all surgeries, patient selection is critical. Niki and colleagues[4] offered limitations on degree of deformity that could be reliably corrected with MDCO and FDL transfer by assessing 25 subjects with stage II flatfoot treated with these procedures. They assessed radiographic correction to determine factors affecting retained alignment. Body mass index was found to not influence longevity of correction. Of 8 radiographic measures on AP and lateral imaging, they identified the lateral talometatarsal angle (LTMT), or Meary's angle, and the tibiocalcaneal angle (TBC) as being affected by MDCO. These were the only parameters to improve postoperatively and showed maintained correction at final follow-up (average of 5.6 years). Cases that were deemed radiographic failures (final follow-up LTMT >20° and TBC >10°), were found to consistently have more severe preoperative deformity. Subjects with LTMT exceeding 25° and TBC exceeding 15° failed to maintain adequate correction. In another study, Guyton and colleagues[11] demonstrated improvement in radiographic arch parameters in a subject population with similar degrees of deformity.

### Plantar pressure

Extensive cadaveric work has investigated the changes in pressure gradients following posterior calcaneal osteotomies. One such study demonstrated that plantar pressures are shifted from the medial forefoot toward the lateral heel following a 1 cm MDCO. Significant decreases in plantar pressure were seen at the first and second metatarsal head, whereas significant increase in pressure was seen at the lateral heel.[12] When combined with an FDL transfer, kinematic studies have demonstrated a more complex shift in plantar pressures and forces. There is a net increase in force transmission in the medial midfoot and forefoot. Additionally, plantar pressure shifted toward the forefoot while the lesser toes were unloaded.[13] Steffensmeier and colleagues[14] studied the impact of MDCO on pressure distributions within the ankle joint using pressure-sensitive film. They demonstrated that 1 cm shifts produced statistically significant changes in pressures within the medial and lateral tibiotalar joint.

### Pain and function

Often paired with FDL transfer, the MDCO has shown to improve pain and function. In a cohort study of 26 subjects, Guyton and colleagues[11] reported great success with pain relief; 91% reported excellent or good pain relief. Twenty-three of 26 subjects reported ability to perform a single leg heel rise, which they all were previously unable to do. Despite this success and documented radiographic correction, nearly all subjects failed to notice a change in foot architecture from an MDCO with FDL transfer. Thus, it is important to openly discuss and counsel patients on postoperative expectations. Schuh and colleagues[13] demonstrated a statistically significant correlation between medial midfoot loading pattern and the American Orthopedic Foot and Ankle Score (AOFAS) score. Isolated MDCO and FDL transfer was studied in the young flatfoot population. Usuelli and colleagues[15] demonstrated postoperative sports participation was higher following surgical correction of early flatfoot than preoperative rates. Thus, limitation in activities of interest should be considered when evaluating patients with early flatfoot deformity. This success has been demonstrated in multiple other studies, although patient populations have not been restricted to isolated MDCO and FDL transfer.[3]

### SUMMARY

The MDCO is a highly useful and efficient tool that should be considered in the algorithm of surgical correction for adult acquired flatfoot deformity. When radiographic and clinical examination determines hindfoot valgus to be a component of the existing deformity, the MDCO has clear benefits. A simple oblique incision with minimal surgical risk is used for the approach. The osteotomy is easy to perform and has a reliable impact on hindfoot valgus, allowing in-depth preoperative planning. The resulting clinical affects include normalizing shifts in plantar pressures, as well as balancing of the pressure distributions in the hindfoot and ankle. Clinically, the MDCO has been shown to decrease pain and improve function. However, because it affects specific components of the flatfoot pathologic condition, this procedure is often needed in combination with other interventions. In more severe cases, it will fail to provide full correction as a stand-alone operation.

### REFERENCES

1. Deland JT. Adult-acquired flatfoot deformity. J Am Acad Orthop Surg 2008;16(7): 399–406. Available at: http://www.ncbi.nlm.nih.gov/pubmed/18611997. Accessed February 12, 2017.

2. Nyska M, Parks BG, Chu IT, et al. The contribution of the medial calcaneal osteotomy to the correction of flatfoot deformities. Foot Ankle Int 2001;22(4):278–82. Available at: http://www.ncbi.nlm.nih.gov/pubmed/11354439. Accessed February 12, 2017.

3. Tellisi N, Lobo M, O'Malley M, et al. Functional outcome after surgical reconstruction of posterior tibial tendon insufficiency in patients under 50 years. Foot Ankle Int 2008;29(12):1179–83.

4. Niki H, Hirano T, Okada H, et al. Outcome of medial displacement calcaneal osteotomy for correction of adult-acquired flatfoot. Foot Ankle Int 2012;33(11): 940–6.

5. Saltzman CL, el-Khoury GY. The hindfoot alignment view. Foot Ankle Int 1995;16(9): 572–6. Available at: http://www.ncbi.nlm.nih.gov/pubmed/8563927. Accessed February 12, 2017.
6. Reilingh ML, Beimers L, Tuijthof GJM, et al. Measuring hindfoot alignment radiographically: the long axial view is more reliable than the hindfoot alignment view. Skeletal Radiol 2010;39(11):1103–8.
7. Conti MS, Ellis SJ, Chan JY, et al. Optimal position of the heel following reconstruction of the stage II adult-acquired flatfoot deformity. Foot Ankle Int 2015; 36(8):919–27.
8. Chan JY, Williams BR, Nair P, et al. The contribution of medializing calcaneal osteotomy on hindfoot alignment in the reconstruction of the stage II adult acquired flatfoot deformity. Foot Ankle Int 2013;34(2):159–66.
9. Feuerstein CA, Weil L Jr, Weil LS Sr, et al. The calcaneal scarf osteotomy: surgical correction of the adult acquired flatfoot deformity and radiographic results. Foot Ankle Spec 2013;6(5):367–71.
10. Greene DL, Thompson MC, Gesink DS, et al. Anatomic study of the medial neurovascular structures in relation to calcaneal osteotomy. Foot Ankle Int 2001;22(7): 569–71. Available at: http://www.ncbi.nlm.nih.gov/pubmed/11503981. Accessed February 12, 2017.
11. Guyton GP, Jeng C, Krieger LE, et al. Flexor digitorum longus transfer and medial displacement calcaneal osteotomy for posterior tibial tendon dysfunction: a middle-term clinical follow-up. Foot Ankle Int 2001;22(8):627–32. Available at: http://www.ncbi.nlm.nih.gov/pubmed/11527022. Accessed February 12, 2017.
12. Hadfield MH, Snyder JW, Liacouras PC, et al. Effects of medializing calcaneal osteotomy on Achilles tendon lengthening and plantar foot pressures. Foot Ankle Int 2003;24(7):523–9. Available at: http://www.ncbi.nlm.nih.gov/pubmed/12921356. Accessed February 12, 2017.
13. Schuh R, Gruber F, Wanivenhaus A, et al. Flexor digitorum longus transfer and medial displacement calcaneal osteotomy for the treatment of stage II posterior tibial tendon dysfunction: kinematic and functional results of fifty one feet. Int Orthop 2013;37(9):1815–20.
14. Steffensmeier SJ, Berbaum KS, Brown TD, et al. Effects of medial and lateral displacement calcaneal osteotomies on tibiotalar joint contact stresses. J Orthop Res 1996;14(6):980–5.
15. Usuelli FG, Di Silvestri CA, D'Ambrosi R, et al. Return to sport activities after medial displacement calcaneal osteotomy and flexor digitorum longus transfer. Knee Surg Sports Traumatol Arthrosc 2016. http://dx.doi.org/10.1007/s00167-016-4360-2.

# Evans Osteotomy Complications

 CrossMark

Marcelo E. Jara, MD

## KEYWORDS

- Plano valgus deformity • Flatfoot deformity • Evans osteotomy • Spastic flatfoot
- Tarsal coalition • Calcaneal Lengthening

## KEY POINTS

- Evans osteotomy has a 3-dimensional effect that renders it irreplaceable in the surgical management of flexible valgus flat foot.
- The complications associated with the technique are of low incidence and are related to patient selection, surgical approach, and correction of foot geometry.
- Nonunion of the osteotomy is infrequent and unrelated to the type of fixation.
- Lateral column overload is a complication related to the magnitude of the correction.
- Achilles tendon lengthening is essential to avoid undercorrection and recurrence of the flat foot.

## INTRODUCTION

In 1975, Evans[1] published his paper on the surgical management of the "calcaneo-valgus deformity" in pediatric patients, pointing out that the deformity was due to the relative shortening of the lateral column of the foot. To achieve correction, it was necessary to "equalize" both columns by performing an osteotomy in the neck of the calcaneus 1.5 cm from the calcaneocuboid joint (CC), where a trapezoidal wedge of tricortical bone taken from the tibia was placed. Although it was considered a success, this first clinical series was not exempt of complications. Sural nerve injury, surgical wound dehiscence, undercorrection, and graft subsidence were described. Given its great power of correction, the osteotomy grew in popularity and its indication extended to other forms of flat foot with similar results and with a low incidence of complications.

Evans osteotomy is indicated in the flexible, painful flat foot that does not respond to conservative treatment and that presents with abduction of the forefoot, calcaneus valgus and dorsolateral peritalar subluxation. The rigid flat foot that does not passively recover its shape is a relative contraindication because in these cases the correction obtained only on the basis of the elongation of the lateral column will be poor, as has also been pointed out in other publications.[2]

A variant of the original technique, the Z-osteotomy performed at the same site, was published in 2008 by Griend[3] to minimize the complications associated with the usual

The author has nothing to disclose.
Orthopaedic Department, Clínica Dávila, Santiago, Chile
*E-mail address:* mjabalos.tmt@gmail.com

Foot Ankle Clin N Am 22 (2017) 573–585
http://dx.doi.org/10.1016/j.fcl.2017.04.006

procedure. Despite a small number of patients (8 feet), no complications were reported, which is consistent with subsequent results.[4,5]

## PATIENT SELECTION

Evans osteotomy is rarely performed in isolation, and in the vast majority of cases it is used in combination with other osteotomies and soft tissue procedures with satisfactory clinical and radiologic results.[6–8]

Proper patient selection is the first measure to minimize complications. With the patient standing, the loss of the plantar arch (**Fig. 1**A), valgus of the calcaneus, and abduction of the forefoot (too many toes sign; see **Fig. 1**B, C) should be identified. The pain in the medial and plantar aspect of the foot is caused by stretching of the soft tissues and spring ligament under the head of the talus, which is usually flexed by the shortening of the gastrosoleus complex. Patients may also experience pain and tenderness in the sinus tarsi by synovitis and impingement of the anterior border of the posterior facet of the calcaneus. The pain may also be located under the tip of the fibula because of the impingement produced by the sustained eversion of the subtalar joint.

The identification of the shortening of the gastrosoleus complex, as mentioned previously, is of vital importance because it is one of the key deforming forces under the foot's morphology, the location of pain and the appearance of late degenerative changes. The shortening will be identified by performing the Silfverskjöld[9] test to define before the osteotomies if an Achilles tendon lengthening or gastrocnemius recession is required. To assess the flexibility of the talonavicular joint and, therefore, the effect of the Evans osteotomy the hindfoot must be reduced with the flexed knee (**Fig. 2**A). The thumb of the same hand holding the calcaneus should rest on

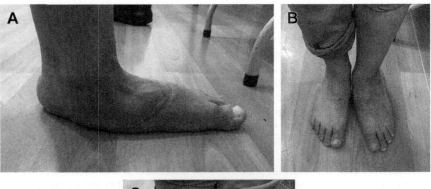

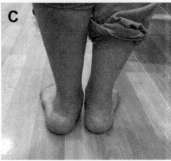

**Fig. 1.** (*A*) Flattening of the longitudinal arch. (*B*) Left forefoot abduction. (*C*) Hindfoot valgus and asymmetrical left forefoot abduction from the rear view (too many toes sign).

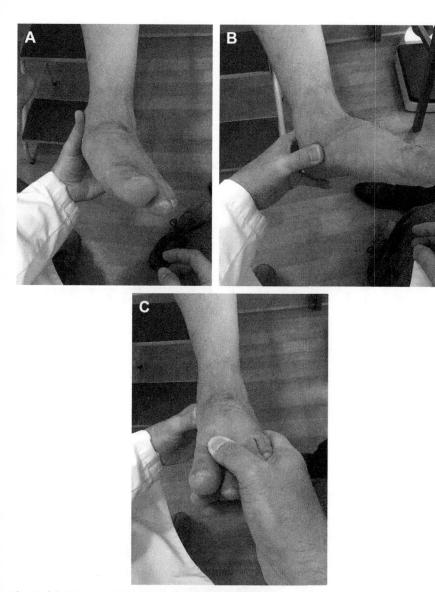

**Fig. 2.** (*A*) Calcaneus in neutral position with flexed knee. (*B*) Thumb holding the medial aspect of the head of the talus. (*C*) The forefoot is reduced from abduction to aligning with the hindfoot and leg.

the medial aspect of the head of the talus (see **Fig. 2**B) while the other hand holds the forefoot and passively reduces it to the position where the head of the talus is completely covered and the forefoot is in line with the heel and the leg.

## COMPLICATIONS

Few publications have focused on the complications associated with the technique and most of them have been described as part of the results of clinical series. The most frequent complications are:

- Nonunion of the osteotomy,
- Dorsal displacement of the anterior calcaneal tuberosity,
- Calcaneocuboid osteoarthritis,

- Lateral foot pain,
- Stress fractures of the fifth metatarsal,
- Loss of calcaneus lengthening,
- Overcorrection,
- Undercorrection,
- Relapse of deformity,
- Injury of sural nerve and peroneal tendons, and
- Invasion of the subtalar joint complex.

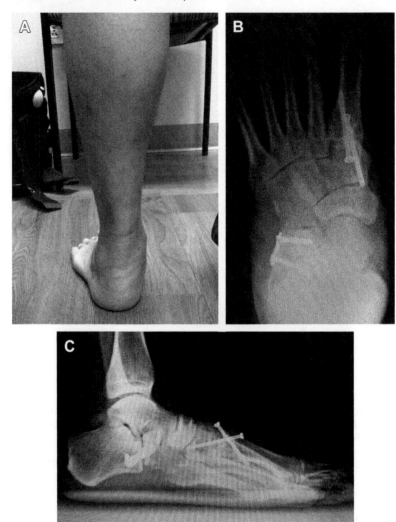

**Fig. 3.** (*A*) A 29-year-old patient, with recurrence of the abduction of the forefoot and lateral pain. (*B*) There is shortening of the lateral column and loss of coverage of the head of the talus. (*C*) Nonunion of the Evans osteotomy with dorsal displacement of the anterior tuberosity of the calcaneus and subluxation of the calcaneocuboid joint. The proximal screw of the plate acted as a rotational axis and the plate acts as a spacer.

## Nonunion of the Osteotomy

In a systematic review, Prissel and Roukis[10] found only 5 studies that met the inclusion criteria (nonunion rate for unfixated isolated Evans osteotomy, follow-up of at least 1 year, and a sample of at least 5 feet). In a total of 73 feet with a mean age of 22 years and an average follow-up of 3.6 years the incidence of nonunion in unfixed Evans osteotomies was 1.4%. Other studies have shown similar incidences as Haeseker and associates,[11] who reported 1 nonunion among 19 patients (5.26%), Zwipp and Rammelt,[12] who reported 1 case in 21 patients (4%), and Hintermann and coworkers,[6] who reported 1 in 19 (5.26%). In all cases revision and bone grafting allowed for consolidation.

Among the factors that influence its low incidence is the rich vascularization of the calcaneus and the press fit of the graft at the site of the osteotomy. Although the mechanism by which the osteotomy exerts its effect is not fully understood, the fact that the foot follows the displacement of the CC joint suggests that the long plantar ligament acts as a pivot, the talonavicular joint as the axis of rotation, and the Spring ligament as hinge (**Fig. 3**). This 3-dimensional movement also allows the peroneus longus tendon to recover its plantar flexor effect on the first metatarsal by retrograde pressing of the graft site.[7,13,14] These changes and the recovery of the windlass mechanism of the plantar fascia increase the bowstring effect that restore the longitudinal arch and increase the stability of the osteotomy.

## Dorsal Displacement of the Anterior Calcaneal Tuberosity

Dorsal subluxation of the anterior tuberosity of the calcaneus (see **Fig. 4E**) is a frequent finding with an incidence ranging from 11.8%[15] to 100%.[16] Although the cause is not fully established, it should in part be because the sustained abduction of the forefoot would produce a shortening of lateral soft tissues that are stretched during lengthening (lateral fascicle of the plantar fascia and aponeurosis of the abductor digiti minimi). Correction would produce a windlass effect under the lateral column squeezing dorsally the anterior process of the calcaneus despite the joint capsule's indemnity. In this process, the long plantar ligament would also participate producing the adduction and plantar flexion of the cuboid as demonstrated by DuMontier and colleagues.[17]

Dunn and Meyer,[18] in a retrospective radiographic study on unfixed osteotomies, demonstrated a significant dorsal displacement until the sixth week followed by spontaneous resolution toward the end of follow-up. The other radiologic parameters as well as clinical results were maintained over time and no patient required further procedures. In 1995, Mosca[19] published transarticular stabilization of the fragment before placing the graft to control its displacement. Wither 1 or 2 Kirshner wires were placed from the cuboid to the proximal calcaneus if subluxation was observed during distraction; however, in both unfixed and fixed patients the results were satisfactory in the long term without any complications. Adams and associates[20] also reported that the fixation of the anterior tuberosity does not significantly reduce the incidence or extent of subluxation and that the correction of abduction does not change in the long term. In all publications, the presence of CC joint arthritis is of low incidence and not always attributable to osteotomy.[1,20]

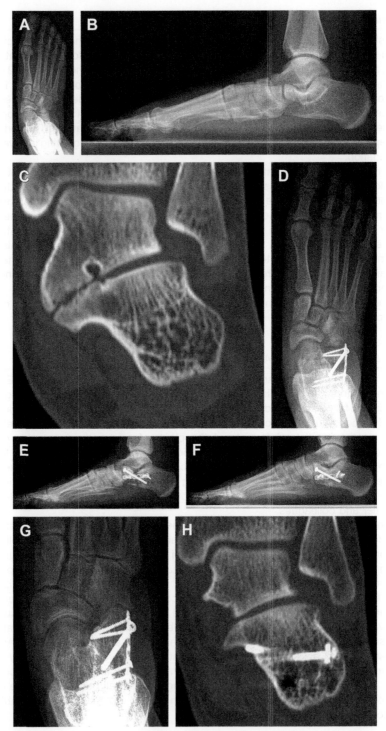

**Fig. 4.** (A) A 15-year-old patient with flat foot valgus and forefoot abduction. (B) Flattening of the plantar arch and C sign, associated with chondral talocalcaneal coalition, which is

*Lateral Pain, Stress Fractures, and Increase Pressure of the Lateral Column*

Several studies have shown that in the flat foot there is a medial displacement of the loads. In a cadaveric model, Oh and colleagues[21] showed an increase of load under the medial column of 21% when the posterior tibial tendon, the inferior interosseous talonavicular ligament, and the spring ligament were removed. Other publications have also shown an increase in the contact surface under the longitudinal arch in both children and adults.[22,23] It has also been shown that abduction of the forefoot produces an increase in calcaneocuboid pressure that would not exceed the limits of physiologic resistance of articular cartilage given the low frequency of CC joint osteoarthritis in patients with long-standing planovalgus deformity.[24] The lengthening of the lateral column is related to the increase of the plantar pressure[15,21,24,25] throughout the column and with the increase of the pressure in the CC joint.[26] This increase in intraarticular pressure has been associated, in turn, with its late degeneration (see **Fig. 4**F,G), with stress fractures of the fifth metatarsal and with the presence of lateral pain up to 11.2% of patients according to Ellis and colleagues.[27] These findings led Cooper and associates[26] to recommend distraction bone block arthrodesis through the CC joint to avoid such complications. However, as other publications have shown,[25,26] in the arthrodesis of the lateral column are more frequent nonunions (11.8%), delayed unions (17.6%), graft stress fractures (17.6%), the residual supination (17.6%), the stress fracture of the fifth metatarsal (5.9%), and the fracture of the screws (5.9%), facts that were not reported in patients undergoing Evans osteotomy. Deland and coworkers[28] further demonstrated that fusion of the lateral column decreases the mobility of the talonavicular joint by 48% and the subtalar joint by 30%, mainly restricting eversion, which contributes to the increase of lateral column pressure. There are no biomechanical studies that indicate an intraarticular pressure threshold associated with the development of CC joint arthritis, although the pressure increases after the osteotomy, its level is not statistically different from the pressure found in the preexisting deformity.[29,30] Because CC joint arthrosis in the planovalgus deformity is an uncommon finding, it is possible to suppose that the lengthening of the lateral column within certain limits does not increase its incidence significantly in the long term, as has been pointed out by several clinical series.[1,4,6,12,19]

In almost all publications, the size of the graft fluctuates between 6 and 12 mm; however, according to results obtained in cadaveric studies,[29] the pressure in the CC joint begins to increase when the graft is greater than 8 mm and increases significantly with respect to a normal foot with grafts greater than 10 mm wide, so that if greater correction is necessary, it is recommended to combine the osteotomy with other complementary procedures.

◄——————————————————————————————

confirmed by computed tomography scan. (*C*) The valgus of the calcaneus is 34°. (*D*) The resection of the bar, Achilles tendon lengthening, and Evans osteotomy were made. (*E*) Elevation of the arch and dorsal displacement of the anterior process of the calcaneus are observed. (*F*) Two years later, the elevation of the arch is maintained but the medial and plantar pain return. (*G*) Correction of lateral column is maintained. Osteophytes appear in the calcaneocuboid joint with no pain. (*H*) The CT scan shows lack of correction of the hindfoot valgus.

### Loss of Calcaneal Lengthening

According to Evans,[1] the sinking of the graft into a too-soft calcaneus is a potential complication that can occur in patients with age-related osteoporosis or in other conditions such as spina bifida. To reduce the risk of loss of correction (see **Fig. 3**A), modifications have been made to the shape of the original osteotomy[3–5] and more stable fixation methods have been developed such as wedge locking plates or titanium wedges to be used in combination with the Z-osteotomy (see **Fig. 5**A,B). The use of plates has a high rate of consolidation, greater load to failure than single screw, better control of the dorsal displacement of the calcaneus, and better maintenance of the length of the lateral column[31]; however, it requires more dissection and its removal may be necessary if there is pain or irritation of the peroneal tendons. Therefore, these modifications should be considered in selected patients because, in the vast majority, the classical technique ensures a sustained correction over time.[6,19,32,33]

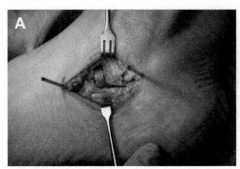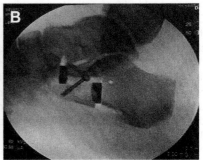

**Fig. 5.** (A) Z-osteotomy with titanium wedges to increase stability. (B) Fixation with a cannulated screw.

### Overcorrection and Recurrence of Deformity

Overcorrection and recurrence are infrequent complications that are associated mainly with flexible flat foot of spastic origin.[34] Although Evans did not recommend the procedure in patients with spasticity, the results of osteotomy combined with other soft tissue procedures in patients with various forms of cerebral palsy have achieved satisfactory results of up to 65% with an incidence of overcorrection of 8.7% and recurrence rate of 15.2%, as reported by Zeifang and colleagues.[34] Although it is not easy to determine the cause of the overcorrection, it has been postulated that the apparent spasticity of the posterior tibial can precipitate its onset.[35]

Cerebral palsy can occur in its spastic form in 85% of cases and less commonly in its dyskinetic variant.[36] Clinically, it adopts the presentation of hemiplegia, diplegia, and spastic quadriplegia. Although the first 2 forms of presentation can walk independently or assisted with some devices, quadriplegic patients rarely present functional gait and their inclusion in this series should be taken with reservations (3 cases; 2 good and 1 relapse).

### Undercorrection

In the adult population, the best procedure for rigid valgus flat foot is the triple arthrodesis[37,38]; however, in the pediatric and adolescent population, the most frequent cause of stiffness is not the posterior tibial tendon insufficiency but tarsal coalitions (see **Fig. 4**). In these cases, the fusions are not desirable because they transfer the stress to the ankle and to the Chopart joint. Evans[1] recognized that the isolated lengthening of the lateral column in calcaneonavicular coalitions relieved pain but was a cause of undercorrection and, according to more recent publications, the persistence of hindfoot valgus is associated with poor outcomes.[39–41] Because the shape of the foot in patients with tarsal coalitions is related not only to the abduction of the forefoot, but also to the structural valgus of the subtalar (see **Fig. 4**C), the correction should consider Achilles tendon lengthening, resection of the bars, lateral column lengthening, and medializing the calcaneal osteotomy to restore the geometry of the foot. Ideally, the preoperative evaluation should include a computed tomography scan to rule out a second coalition present up to 20%, as described by Clarke.[42] The results of resection and subsequent reconstruction are satisfactory if these criteria are incorporated in the treatment of talocalcaneal[43] and calcaneonavicular coalitions.[44]

According to Wilde and associates,[40] some talocalcaneal coalitions are not resectable; however, Mosca and Bevan[43] published a series of 5 patients with unresectable bars and an average 31° of hindfoot valgus, who underwent 9 Evans osteotomies and Achilles tendon lengthening. The mean follow-up duration was 3.7 years (range, 2.0–5.2) and the American Orthopaedic Foot and Ankle Society ankle–hindfoot score for the group improved from 61.3 (range, 58–65) to 90 (range, 84–94). In this series, the maximum postoperative score is 94 because of the rigidity of the subtalar joint owing to the bar.

The explanation of this dissociation between the presence of the bar and the good results of the Evans osteotomy is because the osteotomy does not produce varus movement of the subtalar joint and that the apparent position is due to the effects that occur in the midfoot and forefoot, that is, distal to the site of the talocalcaneal bar, as demonstrated by DuMontier and coworkers in their cadaveric study.[17]

### Injury of Anatomic Structures at Risk

#### Sural nerve and peroneal tendons

Sural nerve injury has been reported with an incidence of 11% according to Thomas and colleagues,[15] whereas the lesion of the peroneal tendon has been reported only occasionally (**Fig. 6**). Anatomic studies have shown that no matter how far from the CC joint is the osteotomy (range, 5–15 mm), always the sural nerve and the peroneus brevis tendon will be found on it, although the peroneus longus tendon will be found at risk if the osteotomy is done less than 10 mm from the joint.

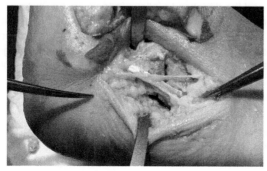

**Fig. 6.** The site of the osteotomy is crossed by the peroneus brevis tendon and by the sural nerve.

## Subtalar joint complex

In an extensive anatomic study performed by Ragab and associates,[45] a total of 1056 calcaneus were examined and it was found that in only 37% the anterior and middle facets were separated, 6% had no anterior facet, and the rest had both facets united. These results coincide with other studies in which the proportion of separated anterior and middle facets is close to only one-third of the population.[46] According to these data, the possibility of avoiding invasion of 1 of the 2 facets during the osteotomy fluctuates between 37% and 44%.[47]

Other points of controversy are as follows: the starting point of the osteotomy and its direction during the cut. The recommendations range between 4 mm according to Trnka and colleagues[48–51] and 1.5 cm according to other publications, including that of Evans.[1] In a cadaveric study in adults Bussewitz and coworkers[47] pointed out that beginning the osteotomy at 1.3 cm from the CC joint and turning slightly from posterolateral to anteromedial, the risk of damaging the sustentaculum tali was reduced, an observation that coincides with that made by Mosca.[19] According to the usual recommendations the osteotomy should be performed parallel to the CC joint; however, Bussewitz and associates[47] showed that in 4 of 10 specimens the sustentaculum tali was included in the osteotomy, which risked its stability.

Evans performed the osteotomy at a greater distance from the CC joint in smaller feet so that, if Bussewitz's observations are correct, many of the osteotomies performed in that first series must have invaded the middle facet; however, as Phillips[32] found in 17 of the 23 original patients, the results were satisfactory at 13 years of mean follow-up.

All these observations are aimed at avoiding incongruities in the subtalar joint and injure both the sustentaculum tali and the anterior calcaneal facet; however, the anterior facet, when it exists, is not supporting the head of the talus but has a plantar–lateral location to it serving more as a site of insertion of the inferior calcaneonavicular ligament than as a true joint.

The structures included in the tarsal tunnel[52] are also under the potential risk of iatrogenic lesions, although there are no publications that report lesions of the flexor hallucis longus tendon or medial plantar nerve in relation to the osteotomy but rather to expansive processes, talocalcaneal coalitions,[53] and nonunions derived from fractures of sustentaculum tali.[54]

## FINAL CONSIDERATIONS

It is remarkable that, although it is an intraarticular osteotomy in most cases, the Evans osteotomy is not associated with the appearance of subtalar osteoarthritis regardless of the site chosen and the direction to follow. Indeed, as the Phillips series[32] shows on Evans's patients in the largest follow-up published to date, Evans osteotomy is a reliable technique in the long term and its association with other procedures chosen on the basis of a thorough physical examination and an adequate imaging study makes it an irreplaceable tool in the management of painful flexible pes planovalgus at all ages.

## REFERENCES

1. Evans D. Calcaneo-valgus deformity. J Bone Joint Surg Br 1975;57(3):270–8.
2. Mahan KT, McGlamry ED. Evans calcaneal osteotomy for flexible pes valgus deformity. A preliminary study. Clin Podiatr Med Surg 1987;4(1):137–51.
3. Griend RV. Lateral column lengthening using a "Z" osteotomy of the calcaneus. Tech Foot Ankle Surg 2008;7(4):257–63.

4. Demetracopoulos C, Nair P, Malzberg A, et al. Outcomes of a stepcut lengthening calcaneal osteotomy for adult-acquired flatfoot deformity. Foot Ankle Int 2015;36(7):749–55.
5. Scott R, Berlet G. Calcaneal Z osteotomy for extra-articular correction of hindfoot valgus. J Foot Ankle Surg 2013;52(3):406–8.
6. Hintermann B, Valderrabano V, Kundert H. Lengthening of the lateral column and reconstruction of the medial soft tissue for treatment of acquired flatfoot deformity associated with insufficiency of the posterior tibial tendon. Foot Ankle Int 1999;20: 622–9.
7. Pomeroy G, Manoli A 2nd. A new operative approach for flatfoot secondary to posterior tibial tendon insufficiency: a preliminary report. Foot Ankle Int 1997; 18(4):206–12.
8. Iossi M, Johnson J, McCormick J, et al. Short-term radiographic analysis of operative correction of adult acquired flatfoot deformity. Foot Ankle Int 2013;34(6): 781–91.
9. Silfversköld N. Reduction of the uncrossed two-joints muscles of the leg to one-joint muscles in spastic conditions. Acta Chir Scand 1924;56:53.
10. Prissel M, Roukis T. Incidence of nonunion of the unfixated, isolated Evans calcaneal osteotomy: a systematic review. J Foot Ankle Surg 2012;51(3):323–5.
11. Haeseker G, Mureau M, Faber F. Lateral column lengthening for acquired adult flatfoot deformity caused by posterior tibial tendon dysfunction stage II: a retrospective comparison of calcaneus osteotomy with calcaneocuboid distraction arthrodesis. J Foot Ankle Surg 2010;49(4):380–4.
12. Zwipp H, Rammelt S. Modified Evans osteotomy for the operative treatment of acquired pes planovalgus. Oper Orthop Traumatol 2006;18(2):182–97.
13. Huang C, Kitaoka H, An K, et al. Biomechanical evaluation of longitudinal arch stability. Foot Ankle 1993;14(6):353–7.
14. Sangeorzan B, Mosca V, Hansen ST Jr. Effect of calcaneal lengthening on relationships among the hindfoot, midfoot, and forefoot. Foot Ankle 1993;14(3): 136–41.
15. Thomas R, Wells B, Garrison R, et al. Preliminary results comparing two methods of lateral column lengthening. Foot Ankle Int 2001;22(2):107–19.
16. Ahn J, Lee H, Kim C, et al. Calcaneocuboid joint subluxation after the calcaneal lengthening procedure in children. Foot Ankle Int 2014;35(7):677–82.
17. DuMontier T, Falicov A, Mosca V, et al. Calcaneal lengthening: investigation of deformity correction in a cadaver flatfoot model. Foot Ankle Int 2005;26(2): 166–70.
18. Dunn S, Meyer J. Displacement of the anterior process of the calcaneus after Evans calcaneal osteotomy. J Foot Ankle Surg 2011;50(4):402–6.
19. Mosca V. Calcaneal lengthening for valgus deformity of the hindfoot. Results in children who had severe, symptomatic flatfoot and skewfoot. J Bone Joint Surg Am 1995;77(4):500–12.
20. Adams S, Simpson A, Pugh L, et al. Calcaneocuboid joint subluxation after calcaneal lengthening for planovalgus foot deformity in children with cerebral palsy. J Pediatr Orthop 2009;29(2):170–4.
21. Oh I, Imhauser C, Choi D, et al. Sensitivity of plantar pressure and talonavicular alignment to lateral column lengthening in flatfoot reconstruction. J Bone Joint Surg Am 2013;95(12):1094–100.
22. Pauk J, Ihnatouski M, Najafi B. Assessing plantar pressure distribution in children with flatfoot arch: application of the Clarke angle. J Am Podiatr Med Assoc 2014; 104(6):622–32.

23. Szczygiel E, Golec E, Golec J, et al. Comparative analysis of distribution on the sole surface of arched feet and flat feet. Przegl Lek 2008;65(1):4–7.
24. Ellis S, Yu J, Johnson A, et al. Plantar pressures in patients with and without lateral foot pain after lateral column lengthening. J Bone Joint Surg Am 2010;92(1): 81–91.
25. Tien T, Parks B, Guyton G. Plantar pressures in the forefoot after lateral column lengthening: a cadaver study comparing the Evans osteotomy and calcaneocuboid fusion. Foot Ankle Int 2005;26(7):520–5.
26. Cooper P, Nowak M, Shaer J. Calcaneocuboid joint pressures with lateral column lengthening (Evans) procedure. Foot Ankle Int 1997;18(4):199–205.
27. Ellis S, Williams B, Garg R, et al. Incidence of plantar lateral foot pain before and after the use of trial metal wedges in lateral column lengthening. Foot Ankle Int 2011;32(7):665–73.
28. Deland J, Otis J, Lee K, et al. Lateral column lengthening with calcaneocuboid fusion: range of motion in the triple joint complex. Foot Ankle Int 1995;16(11): 729–33.
29. Momberger N, Morgan J, Bachus K, et al. Calcaneocuboid joint pressure after lateral column lengthening in a cadaveric planovalgus deformity model. Foot Ankle Int 2000;21(9):730–5.
30. Dayton P, Prins DB, Smith DE, et al. Effectiveness of a locking plate in preserving midcalcaneal length and positional outcome after Evans calcaneal osteotomy: a retrospective pilot study. J Foot Ankle Surg 2013;52(6):710–3.
31. Protzman N, Wobst G, Storts E, et al. Mid-calcaneal length after Evans calcaneal osteotomy: a retrospective comparison of wedge locking plates and tricortical allograft wedges. J Foot Ankle Surg 2015;54(5):900–4.
32. Phillips GE. A review of elongation of os calcis for flat feet. J Bone Joint Surg Br 1983;65(1):15–8.
33. Davitt J, Morgan J. Stress fracture of the fifth metatarsal after Evans' calcaneal osteotomy: a report of two cases. Foot Ankle Int 1998t;19(10):710–2.
34. Zeifang F, Breusch SJ, Döderlein L. Evans calcaneal lengthening procedure for spastic flexible flatfoot in 32 patients (46 feet) with a followup of 3 to 9 years. Foot Ankle Int 2006;27(7):500–7.
35. Bleck E. Management of the lower extremities in children who have cerebral palsy. J Bone Joint Surg Am 1990;72(1):140–4.
36. Stanley F, Blair E, Alberman E. Cerebral palsies: epidemiology and causal pathways. Clinics in developmental medicine. London: Mac–Keith Press; 2000. p. 151.
37. Pell R, Myerson M, Schon L. Clinical outcome after primary triple arthrodesis. J Bone Joint Surg Am 2000;82(1):47–57.
38. Horton G, Olney B. Triple arthrodesis with lateral column lengthening for treatment of severe planovalgus deformity. Foot Ankle Int 1995;16(7):395–400.
39. Luhmann S, Schoenecker P. Symptomatic talocalcaneal coalition resection: indications and results. J Pediatr Orthop 1998;18:748–54.
40. Wilde P, Torode I, Dickens D, et al. Resection for symptomatic talocalcaneal coalition. J Bone Joint Surg Br 1994;76:797–801.
41. Westberry D, Davids J, Oros W. Surgical management of symptomatic talocalcaneal coalitions by resection of the sustentaculum tali. J Pediatr Orthop 2003;23: 493–7.
42. Clarke D. Multiple tarsal coalitions in the same foot. J Pediatr Orthop 1997;17: 777–80.

43. Mosca V, Bevan W. Talocalcaneal tarsal coalitions and the calcaneal lengthening osteotomy: the role of deformity correction. J Bone Joint Surg Am 2012;94(17): 1584–94.
44. Quinn E, Peterson K, Hyer C. Calcaneonavicular coalition resection with pes planovalgus reconstruction. J Foot Ankle Surg 2016;55(3):578–82.
45. Ragab A, Stewart S, Cooperman D. Implications of subtalar joint anatomic variation in calcaneal lengthening osteotomy. J Pediatr Orthop 2003;23(1):79–83.
46. Bunning P, Barnett C. A comparison of adult and foetal talocalcaneal articulations. J Anat 1965;99:71–6.
47. Bussewitz B, DeVries J, Hyer C. Evans osteotomy and risk to subtalar joint articular facets and sustentaculum tali: a cadaver study. J Foot Ankle Surg 2013; 52(5):594–7.
48. Trnka H, Easley M, Myerson M. The role of calcaneal osteotomies for correction of adult flatfoot. Clin Orthop Relat Res 1999;(365):50–64.
49. Lombardi C, Dennis L, Connolly F, et al. Talonavicular joint arthrodesis and Evans calcaneal osteotomy for treatment of posterior tibial tendon dysfunction. J Foot Ankle Surg 1999;38:116–22.
50. Weinraub G, Heilala M. Adult flatfoot/posterior tibial tendon dysfunction: outcomes analysis of surgical treatment utilizing an algorithmic approach. J Foot Ankle Surg 2000;39:359–64.
51. Golano P, Fariñas O, Sáenz I. The anatomy of the navicular and periarticular structures. Foot Ankle Clin 2004;9(1):1–23.
52. Raines R, Brage M. Evans osteotomy in the adult foot: an anatomic study of structures at risk. Foot Ankle Int 1998;19(11):743–7.
53. Lam S. Tarsal tunnel syndrome. J Bone Joint Surg Br 1967;49(1):87–92.
54. Myerson MS, Berger BI. Nonunion of a fracture of the sustentaculum tali causing a tarsal tunnel syndrome: a case report. Foot Ankle Int 1995;16:740–2.

# Is This My Ankle or My Foot?

William Hodges Davis, MD

## KEYWORDS

- Pathologic flatfoot • Valgus deformity • Degenerative ankle disease • Ankle arthritis

## KEY POINTS

- Traditional thinking has suggested that pathologic flatfoot is a continuum.
- The patients who present with valgus deformity at the ankle (with and without end-stage arthritis) most often do not have a concomitant flatfoot.
- As we continue to progress in our treatment of degenerative ankle disease with valgus deformity, it is imperative for us to embrace this deformity as the end stage in multidirectional global instability.

## INTRODUCTION

The understanding of the complexities of the adult acquired pathologic flatfoot has undergone serious evolution in the past 30 years; from a secure feeling that the process began and ended with failure of the posterior tibial tendon[1] to a greater understanding of the subtleties of what causes the different presentations and drives successful treatment. In addition, as the treatment of ankle arthritis evolves from fusion to ankle replacement, the need for answers for the very difficult patient with valgus degenerative ankle disease begs a look at what causes this form of flatfoot. The following question is posed in this article: is there a subset of patients with "flatfoot" that has little to do with the foot and is all about the ankle?

Traditional thinking has suggested that pathologic flatfoot is a continuum. In the classic article by Johnson and Strom,[2] it was suggested that the so-called "Posterior Tibial Tendon Insufficiency" could be broken into 3 clinical stages, beginning with stage 1 (Johnson and Strom[2]), which is no more than tendonitis. These patients most often have preexisting symmetric congenital flatfoot before presenting. Stage 2 describes a well-known patient with progressive asymmetry in valgus collapse

Disclosure: Products shown in x-rays. Wright Medical: Consulting, Royalties, Research support.
OrthoCarolina Foot and Ankle Institute, 2001 Vail Avenue, Charlotte, NC 28207, USA
E-mail address: hodges.davis@orthocarolina.com

with retained motion in the hindfoot. Stage 3 is felt to be a "progressed stage 2" with resultant degeneration and fixed asymmetric planovalgus deformity. Myerson and then Bluman[3–5] felt that if the progression of the valgus collapse remains unchecked, then the ankle is affected. The addition of stage 4 to include those patients who have valgus ankle collapse has begged the question, is grade 4 really a progression of grade 2 or 3? Smith and Bluman[6] felt this was the case when they wrote " Most patients with stage IV AAFD (Adult Acquired Flatfoot Deformity) have progressed through stage III disease, although a subset of patients develop valgus talar tilt without a rigid flatfoot deformity, suggesting a possible progression directly from stage II to stage IV."

Our experience is in many ways the opposite. The patients who present with valgus deformity at the ankle (with and without end-stage arthritis) most often do not have a concomitant flatfoot. The common history is ankle sprains (recurring or a single significant event). The presentation is with a complaint of a progressive "flatfoot." The symptomatic side is most often unilateral but can be bilateral. These patients appear to have an entirely ankle-derived flatfoot. Although this observation flies in the face of the traditional thinking, it has been observed before by other clinicians.

## DELTOID ANATOMY

The superficial deltoid has been described in 4 consistent fascicles.[7] The anterior fascicles (tibionavicular ligament, tibiospring ligament) tend to be thicker and cross 2 joints. The direct medial (tibiocalcaneal ligament) and posterior (posterior tibiotalar ligament) may be less thick. The superficial deltoid resists valgus deformity (**Fig. 1**). The deep deltoid crosses 1 joint (tibiotalar) and prevents malrotation. In the severe valgus "tilted ankle," both the deep and superficial are involved. The extent is difficult to ascertain by standing radiographs.

## LITERATURE OBSERVATIONS

Hinterman and his group[8–11] have described this condition in a discussion about medial instability. In the Hinterman classification, the progression of the medial instability goes from minimal instability symptoms with giving way to the condition that is seen as end stage, with a resultant flatfoot and even an insufficient posterior tibialis tendon[8] (**Table 1**). The grade III and IV in the medial ankle instability classification truly describes the end stage patient that is confused for a grade IV AAFD.

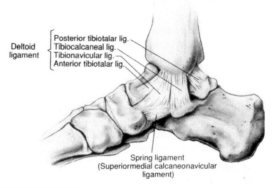

Deltoid ligament
{ Posterior tibiotalar lig.
  Tibiocalcaneal lig.
  Tibionavicular lig.
  Anterior tibiotalar lig.

Spring ligament
(Superiormedial calcaneonavicular ligament)

**Fig. 1.** Deltoid ligament anatomy.

**Table 1**
The Hinterman classification of medial ankle instability: type III and IV are descriptions of the Myerson Grade IV flatfoot in many ways

| | | | Clinical Classification (Type I–IV) | | | |
|---|---|---|---|---|---|---|
| | Giving Way | Hindfoot Valgus | Medial Ankle Pain | Anterolateral Ankle Pain | Posterior Tibialis Tendon Deficiency | Heel Variation |
| Type I | + | + | + | (+) | ... | Yes |
| Type II | ++ | + | +++ | (+) | ... | Yes |
| Type III | +++ | ++ | +++ | + | + | None |
| Type IV | ++++ | +++ | ++++ | ++ | ++ | None |

+, levels of positive findings.

This description does not take into account a multidirectional instability that includes medial and lateral ligaments as well as syndesmotic instability that can be seen early and late in these patients' history.[12,13] This Swiss group has published several articles that have analyzed the medial side of the ankle anatomically, clinically, and described treatment in the acute and subacute settings.[8,10,11] It is in the chronic setting that the confusion in the classifications of type III and IV medial ankle and AAFD stage IV occurs.

**Table 2**
The RAM classification of flatfoot deformities

| | The RAM Classification | | |
|---|---|---|---|
| | Rearfoot | Ankle | Midfoot |
| Ia | Tenosynovitis of posterior tibialis tendon (PTT) | Neutral alignment | Neutral alignment |
| Ib | PTT tendonitis without deformity | Mild valgus (<5°) | Mild flexible midfoot supination |
| IIa | Flexible planovalgus (<40% talar uncoverage, <30° Meary angle, incongruency angle 20° to 45°) | Valgus with deltoid insufficiency (no arthritis) | Midfoot supination without radiographic instability |
| IIb | Flexible planovalgus (>40% talar uncoverage, >30° Meary angle, incongruency angle >45°) | Valgus with deltoid insufficiency with tibiotalar arthritis | Midfoot supination with midfoot instability—no arthritis |
| IIIa | Fixed/arthritic planovalgus (<40% talar uncoverage, <30° Meary angle, incongruency angle 20° to 45°) | Valgus secondary to bone loss in the lateral tibial plafond (deltoid normal) | Arthritic changes isolated to medial column (navicular-medial cuneiform or first Tarsometatarsal Joint joints) |
| IIIb | Fixed/arthritic planovalgus (>40% talar uncoverage, >30° Meary angle, incongruency angle >45°) —not correctable through triple arthrodesis | Valgus secondary to bone loss in the lateral tibial plafond and with deltoid insufficiency | Medial and middle column midfoot arthritic changes (usually with supination and/or abduction of the midfoot) |

Steve Raiken and his group[14] have described the Rearfoot, Ankle, Midfoot (RAM) classification (**Table 2.**) This classification is an attempt to subclassify deformity at the anatomic area that is most affected. The ankle portion of this classification mirrors the thought that valgus and subsequent valgus deformity in the hindfoot can be solely related to ankle pathology, both instability and degeneration. A continued attempt to tie this ankle classification to the hindfoot classification can be confusing, but highlights the complexity of these deformities. The investigators do not give

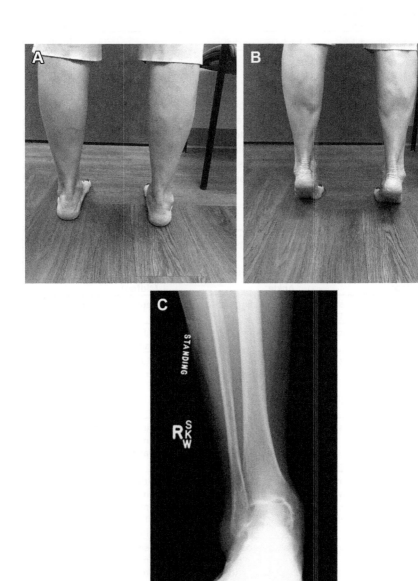

**Fig. 2.** (A) asymmetric flatfoot in patient with multidirectional instability after multiple ankle sprains (B) becomes symmetric with toe raise. (C) Standing radiograph showing valgus collapse.

clinical or radiographic criteria to determine in which deformities the deltoid remains intact. This would be helpful to guide treatment and continues to be a challenge in treatment algorithms for valgus ankle deformity.

Don Bohay and John Anderson[15] have described a patient group that will have a normal foot after an ankle fusion for valgus degenerative ankle. The description is of a derotation of the talus into mortise. The hindfoot collapse is corrected as the ankle is stabilized. This is a clinical scenario that also can be reproduced in the valgus degenerative ankle in a semiconstrained ankle replacement.

## CLINICAL OBSERVATIONS
### *Valgus Ankle with Multidirectional Instability and a Normal Foot*

This patient group has a history that is consistent with multidirectional instability, and is seen more often in athletically active men and women with a history of multiple ankle sprains. Standing examination reveals an asymmetric "too many toes" sign (**Fig. 2**).

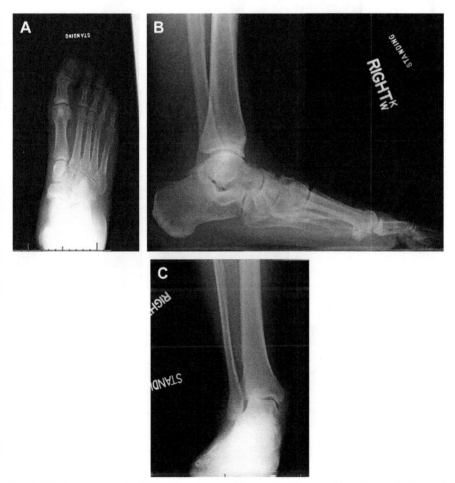

**Fig. 3.** (*A*) Anteroposterior (AP) view of normal foot with valgus ankle collapse. (*B*) Lateral. (*C*) Valgus ankle collapse.

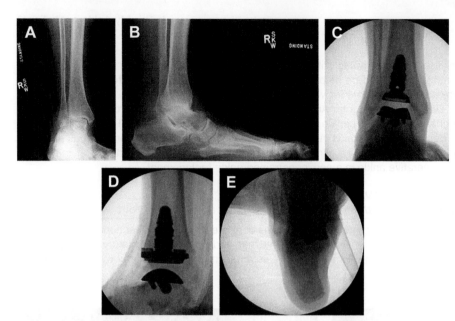

**Fig. 4.** (*A*) Valgus tilted degenerative ankle. (*B*) Normal to cavus foot. (*C*) Intraoperative total ankle replacement (TAR) AP. (*D*) Intraoperative TAR lateral. (*E*) Intraoperative axial view showing varus heel.

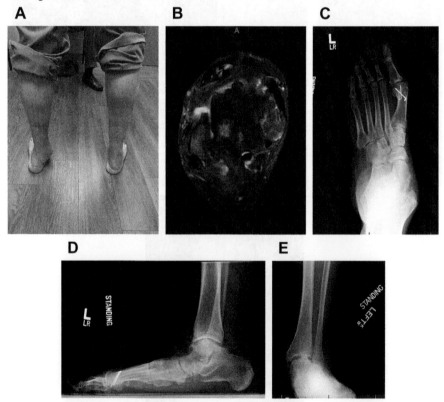

**Fig. 5.** Progressive flatfoot after chronic deltoid instability. Posterior tibial tendon is normal. (*A*) Clinical picture showing collapse. (*B*) MRI showing posterior tibial tendon intact. (*C*) AP foot with minimal talonavicular joint (TN) instability. (*D*) Lateral foot with navicular cuneiform joint (NC) collapse, valgus ankle collapse. (*E*) AP view of the ankle showing Valgus degenerative collapse.

Often rising on the toes recreates the arch. The standing ankle films show the tilted ankle with a normal foot. This patient group often presents with pain from degeneration and the foot remains stable and normal (**Fig. 3**). In the most advanced cases, the degenerative changes are end stage and when the ankle is corrected the foot is truly neutral (**Fig. 4**). Derotating the talus in the mortise does not result in complete correction of the compensatory heel valgus, but it will correct most of the transverse tarsal deformity.

### Valgus Ankle with Unstable Progressive Flatfoot

This patient group fits the more traditional progressive collapse theory except the posterior tibial tendon is most often normal. The flatfoot follows the ankle (**Fig. 5**). These patients tend to have a more complete deltoid tear that makes the reconstruction much more complex. The flatfoot can be more of a sign of the severity of the deltoid instability than the cause of the instability (**Fig. 6**).

### Valgus Ankle with a True Degenerative or a Fused Hindfoot Flatfoot

It is these patients who make one believe that the ankle symptoms are secondary to the progressive rigid flatfoot (**Fig. 7**). The degree of rigid subtalar lateral subluxation, transverse tarsal collapse, fixed compensatory forefoot varus, subfibular impingement with even fibular attritional fractures and valgus degenerative disease of the

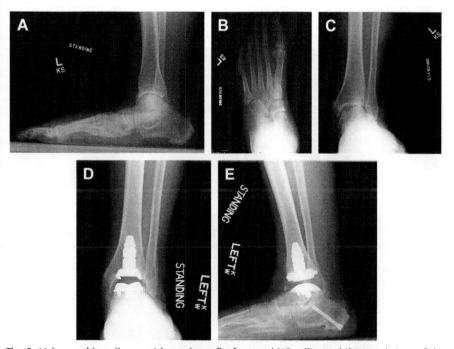

**Fig. 6.** Valgus ankle collapse with resultant flatfoot and NC collapse. (*A*) Lateral view of the foot with NC collapse. (*B*) AP view of the foot with no TN instability. (*C*) Valgus collapse at the ankle. (*D*) AP ankle after ankle replacement with mild residual valgus. (*E*) Lateral of postoperative ankle replacement with medial displacement osteotomy of the calcaneus needed to correct secondary heel valgus.

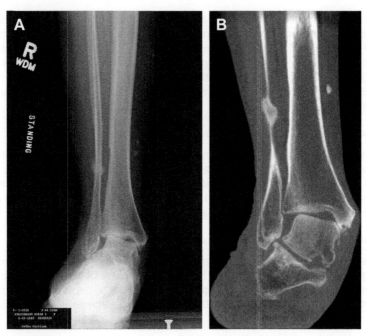

**Fig. 7.** Degenerative flatfoot with valgus collapse and fibula fracture. (*A*) AP ankle. (*B*) Computed tomography scan.

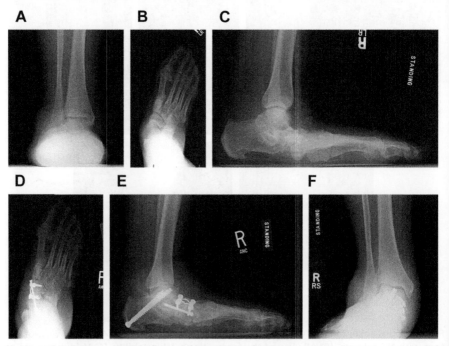

**Fig. 8.** Valgus ankle collapse after hindfoot fusion. (*A*) Preoperative AP ankle with no deltoid instability. (*B*) AP foot with peritalar subluxation. (*C*) Lateral of the foot with TN collapse. (*D*) AP postoperative TN and subtalar fusion. (*E*) Lateral after hindfoot fusion. (*F*) After hindfoot fusion resultant valgus ankle collapse.

ankle is an almost unsolvable problem. An additional scenario that fits in this category is a patient with degenerative planovalgus foot that is stabilized with a hindfoot fusion that develops the valgus degenerative ankle that suggests deltoid insufficiency (**Fig. 8**).

## SUMMARY

The traditional concept of the valgus, tilted ankle as a progression of the classic Johnson and Strom grade 2 or 3 AAFD is at best a small subset of patients that show symptomatic deltoid instability. As we continue to progress in our treatment of degenerative ankle disease with valgus deformity, it is imperative for us to embrace this deformity as the end stage in multidirectional global instability. What remains in question is why a neutral or varus foot would collapse into valgus and not varus? What patient should have early reconstruction to prevent valgus collapse? What is the role of the real but subtle syndesmotic instability in this patient population? The answers will come with careful clinical examination that delineates the different subsets in this difficult ankle disorder.

## REFERENCES

1. Mann RA, Thompson FM. Rupture of the posterior tibial tendon causing flatfoot. J Bone Joint Surg Am 1985;67(4):556–61.
2. Johnson KA, Strom DE. Tinialis posterior tendon dysfunction. Clin Orthop Relat Res 1989;(239):196–203.
3. Bluman EM, Myerson MS. Stage IV posterior tibial tendon rupture. Foot Ankle Clin 2007;12(2):341–62.
4. Bluman EM, Title CI, Myerson MS. Posterior tibial tendon rupture: a refined classification system. Foot Ankle Clin 2007;12(2):233–49.
5. Myerson MS. Adult acquired flatfoot deformity: treatment of dysfunction of the posterior tibial tendon. Instr Course Lect 1997;46:393–405.
6. Smith JT, Bluman EM. Update on stage IV acquired adult flat foot disorder when the deltoid ligament becomes dysfunctional. Foot Ankle Clin 2012;17(2):351–60.
7. Davis WH, Sobel M, Dicarlo EF, et al. Gross, histologic and microvascular anatomy and biomechanical testing of the spring ligament complex. Foot Ankle Int 1996;17(2):95–102.
8. Barg A, Knupp M, Hinterman B. Posttraumatic medial ankle instability. German Trauma Journal 2013;36(1):58–63.
9. Hinterman B. Medial ankle instability. Foot Ankle Clin 2003;8(4):723–38.
10. Hinterman B, Knupp M, Pagenstert GI. Deltoid ligament injuries: diagnosis and management. Foot Ankle Clin 2006;11(3):625–37.
11. Hinterman B, Valderrabano V, Boss A, et al. Medial ankle instability: an exploratory, prospective study of fifty-two cases. Am J Sports Med 2004;32(1):183–90.
12. Crim JR, Beals TC, Nickisch F, et al. Deltoid ligament abnormalities in chronic lateral ligament instability. Foot Ankle Int 2011;32(9):873–8.
13. Jackson JB, Youngblood S, Anderson RB, et al. Gllobal ankle instability: clinical and functional assessment at average 26 month follow-up. Revista da ABTPé 2015;9(1):1–5.
14. Raiken SM, Winters BS, Daniel JN. The RAM classification: a novel, systematic approach to the adult-acquired flatfoot. Foot Ankle Clin 2012;17(2):169–81.
15. Bohay DR, Anderson JG. Stage IV posterior tibialis tendon insufficiency: the tilted ankle. Foot Ankle Clin 2003;8:619–36.

# Overcorrected Flatfoot Reconstruction

Todd A. Irwin, MD

## KEYWORDS

- Flatfoot • Overcorrection • Treatment • Cavovarus
- Posterior tibial tendon dysfunction

## KEY POINTS

- The overcorrected flatfoot reconstruction, although less common than undercorrection, is a complex problem that is challenging to treat.
- A thorough evaluation, including the details of the index operation, is important in determining the cause of the patient's symptoms, which often resemble the cavovarus foot condition.
- Operative management of the overcorrected flatfoot should focus on the patient's specific symptoms and may not require complete reversal of the previous flatfoot correction.
- Combining osteotomies of the calcaneus, midfoot, and forefoot with soft tissue procedures may be sufficient for most revision cases.
- More severe or rigid deformities may require realignment hindfoot and/or midfoot arthrodesis.

## INTRODUCTION

Treatment of the adult acquired flatfoot deformity (AAFD) has significantly evolved over the previous 20 to 30 years. Originally described as failure of the posterior tibial tendon, the concept of posterior tibial tendon dysfunction has persisted and been the topic of multiple studies.[1-3] Johnson and Strom[1] described their classification in 1989, which was later modified by Myerson[4] in 1997. Since that time, the complexity of the AAFD has been studied extensively and is currently better understood.[5-10] However, there is still significant debate regarding the appropriate reconstruction methods. As with all surgical procedures, complications and adverse outcomes can occur when complex reconstruction is performed. This article examines the clinical scenario of an overcorrected flatfoot deformity, how this occurs, and what treatment options are available.

Disclosure Statement: The author has nothing to disclose.
OrthoCarolina Foot and Ankle Institute, 2001 Vail Avenue, Suite 200B, Charlotte, NC 28207, USA
E-mail address: toddairwin@gmail.com

Foot Ankle Clin N Am 22 (2017) 597–611
http://dx.doi.org/10.1016/j.fcl.2017.04.004
1083-7515/17/© 2017 Elsevier Inc. All rights reserved.

foot.theclinics.com

## PATIENT EVALUATION OVERVIEW

Although overcorrection is a recognized complication after flatfoot reconstruction, undercorrection is significantly more common than overcorrection. For more information on undercorrection see Kenneth J. Hunt and Ryan P. Farmer's article, "The Undercorrected Flatfoot Reconstruction," in this issue. AAFD is a complex deformity with multiple clinical components that are interrelated. To better understand what occurs when overcorrection happens it is helpful to break down the physiologic components of the flatfoot deformity (**Box 1**).

Analyzing the treatment of each of the physiologic components outlined in **Box 1** helps to recognize which components are overcorrected. Surgical treatment of AAFD needs to be individualized for each patient and is typically based on the stage of the deformity. Because most patients undergoing surgical correction for AAFD are in the flexible stage II or rigid stage III categories, this article focuses on those two clinical scenarios. The first step in treating the overcorrected patient is to understand what exactly was done during the index procedure. Taking a thorough history and performing a careful physical examination is paramount to understanding the patient's complaint. If possible, reviewing and obtaining the operative report from the index procedure provides important information. Often a patient with an overcorrected flatfoot describes symptoms and has signs similar to the cavovarus foot. As with the patient with AAFD, however, it is similarly important to not oversimplify this clinical scenario and to individualize the treatment of patients with an overcorrected flatfoot. Standing foot (anteroposterior, lateral, and oblique) and ankle (anteroposterior and mortise) radiographs should be reviewed and compared with the patient's preoperative radiographs if available. Comparison views to the contralateral side help to determine the amount of relative deformity. It is important to remember to evaluate the ankle joint radiographically in addition to the foot to assess talar tilt as a possible cause of the deformity. Hindfoot alignment views are also important to determine the amount of hindfoot varus and for comparison with the nonoperative side (**Fig. 1**).[11] Advanced imaging, such as a computed tomography (CT) scan or MRI, is obtained depending on the patient's complaint, although it is often not necessary. CT scan is useful to determine presence of nonunion or arthritic changes as causes of the patient's pain. Weightbearing CT scans have become more available in recent years, which may help to further evaluate hindfoot alignment or possible areas of bone impingement

---

**Box 1**
**Physiologic components of the adult acquired flatfoot deformity**

Insufficiency of the posterior tibial tendon with associated degeneration

Stress/strain on the deltoid-spring ligament complex

Stress/strain on the subtalar joint and transverse tarsal joint capsules

Progressive hindfoot valgus and abduction through the transverse tarsal joints

Plantar collapse of the talar head with associated rotation of the subtalar joint

Shortening of the gastrocnemius-soleus complex and/or Achilles tendon

Possible medial column collapse through naviculocuneiform and/or tarsometatarsal joint

Overpull of the peroneus brevis with possible contracture

Forefoot supination deformity to accommodate foot position and achieve plantigrade foot

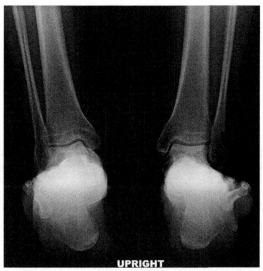

**Fig. 1.** Hindfoot alignment radiograph showing a varus heel posture on the left after flat-foot reconstruction, compared with normal hindfoot alignment on right.

as a result of the previous operation.[12] MRI is useful to determine presence of tendon pathology or bone edema as a cause of the patient's pain.

## NONOPERATIVE TREATMENT OPTIONS

The patient with an overcorrected flatfoot likely presents with symptoms similar to an idiopathic cavovarus foot. Common complaints include lateral foot pain, stiffness, decreased range of motion (typically lack of eversion), plantar forefoot pain, possible lateral ankle instability, and/or lateral ankle pain.[9,13–18] Determining the patient's chief complaint is essential to determine the appropriate intervention.

For lateral foot or plantar forefoot pain, simple offloading treatments may be effective. Isolated first metatarsal head and/or sesamoid pain is treated with an offloading insert, such as a dancer's pad. Lateral heel posting with or without a recessed first ray may be effective for lateral foot pain from overload. This offloading can often be achieved with simple commercially available pads or inserts. For more significant deformity, or if simple pads and reliefs are not effective, bilateral custom orthotics are considered.

For lateral ankle instability, bracing is effective. Commercially available lace-up type braces often minimize the instability episodes, and possibly improve the discomfort. For more significant deformity, a custom brace, such as a short-articulating ankle-foot-orthosis, may be effective. If the patient's complaint is related to stiffness, decreased range of motion, ankle instability episodes, or tendon-related pathology, a trial of physical therapy is a reasonable consideration. Finally, selective corticosteroid injections are used as a diagnostic tool to determine whether specific joints are the source of pain, and temporary symptomatic relief.

## OPERATIVE TREATMENT OPTIONS

When a patient has failed conservative treatment, operative intervention is warranted. Correlating the patient's symptoms with the procedures performed during the index operation helps with preoperative planning. The combination of procedures performed for the initial flatfoot reconstruction ultimately leads to the overcorrected situation; however, the patient's symptoms may be more or less related to only certain procedures performed. As such, the entire flatfoot reconstruction may not have to be undone to appropriately treat the patient's symptoms. Therefore, it is helpful to examine potential overcorrection of each component of a flatfoot reconstruction, and the associated surgical correction.

## GASTROCNEMIUS RECESSION/TENDO-ACHILLES LENGTHENING

A tight gastrocnemius-soleus complex and/or Achilles tendon is a hallmark of AAFD. Most patients who undergo flatfoot reconstruction receive either a gastrocnemius recession or a tendo-Achilles lengthening procedure.[19–21] Theoretically, an overlengthening of the gastrocnemius-soleus-Achilles complex is possible. If present, this could lead to weakness with plantarflexion, and/or possibly a calcaneus gait. The gastrocnemius recession procedure rarely leads to overlengthening.[19] An aggressive tendo-Achilles lengthening, however, can lead to weakness with plantarflexion, although this is uncommon.[9] If present, surgical treatment is rarely indicated, because physical therapy should provide sufficient improvement in strength.

## FLEXOR DIGITORUM LONGUS TENDON TRANSFER

In the presence of an insufficient posterior tibial tendon, the flexor digitorum longus is the most common tendon used for transfer.[6,7,9,10,19,21,22] As with any tendon transfer, achieving the appropriate tension can be difficult to discern.[2,23] Overtightening of the flexor digitorum longus tendon transfer is possible but uncommon because the musculotendinous unit tends to stretch and the tendon can adapt during the early postoperative period.[24] Patients may complain of stiffness, specifically with lack of eversion.[9] Lack of excursion of the transferred tendon is another concern, which could lead to decreased function.[23] Physical therapy should be maximized to increase coronal plane hindfoot range of motion. Theoretically, tenolysis of the transferred tendon with or without Z-lengthening could be considered in a revision situation; however, the need for this is rare.

## MEDIAL DISPLACEMENT CALCANEAL OSTEOTOMY

The medial displacement calcaneal osteotomy (MDCO) is a common procedure to address the hindfoot valgus component of AAFD.[7,9,10,13,19–22,25–27] Biomechanical and clinical studies have evaluated how much translation is appropriate when this procedure is performed.[27–29] Chan and colleagues[27] correlated the amount of translation performed during the MDCO procedure with the hindfoot moment arm as measured with a hindfoot alignment view and found a linear relationship. In addition, some surgeons attempt to not only medially translate but also inferiorly translate the posterior tuberosity to effectively increase the calcaneal pitch (**Fig. 2**). Excessive medial translation, inferior translation, or both can effectively alter the moment arm of the longitudinal alignment of the hindfoot into a varus posture (**Fig. 3**).[8] Conti and colleagues[28] correlated postoperative hindfoot alignment with patient outcomes and found mild radiographic varus (>0–5 mm varus on hindfoot alignment view) was associated with greatest clinical outcomes. Importantly, 20 of their subjects had moderate varus radiographically (>5 mm varus), which was associated with less improvement in symptoms compared with mild varus or residual valgus. The authors also discussed the difference between clinical varus and radiographic varus. They found that a straight heel

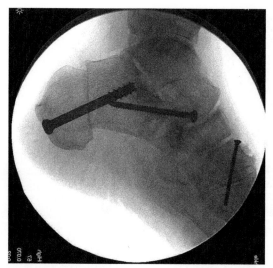

**Fig. 2.** Intraoperative fluoroscopic radiograph showing inferior translation of the calcaneal tuberosity as part of the MDCO portion of the flatfoot reconstruction.

on standing clinical view correlated with mild radiographic varus and the most favorable clinical outcomes (**Fig. 4**).[28]

If either excessive medial translation or inferior translation is determined, a revision calcaneal osteotomy is indicated (**Fig. 5** for case example). As in the cavovarus foot condition, options for a lateralizing calcaneal osteotomy include pure closing wedge osteotomies (Dwyer vs Z-type), lateral translational osteotomies, or a combination of both.[30–33] Care should be taken when performing this osteotomy because of the risk of tibial nerve palsy, which has been reported to be 34%.[33,34] Potential contributing factors to this increased risk are type of osteotomy, location of the osteotomy, and amount of lateral translation performed.[33,35] It is unclear if this risk is minimized in the setting of correcting too much previous medial translation. However, because of possible scar tissue or bone remodeling at the osteotomy site in this revision situation, extra caution should be maintained. If a standard oblique closing wedge

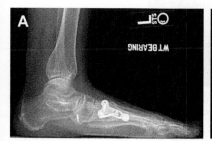
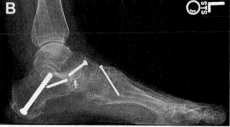

**Fig. 3.** Preoperative lateral foot radiograph (*A*) and 1.5-year postoperative lateral foot radiograph (*B*) after revision flatfoot reconstruction including MDCO, lateral column lengthening (LCL), and Cotton osteotomy through a previously fused first tarsometatarsal joint. Note the increased calcaneal pitch after inferior translation of the posterior calcaneal tuberosity, and the nonunion through the LCL with associated broken screw.

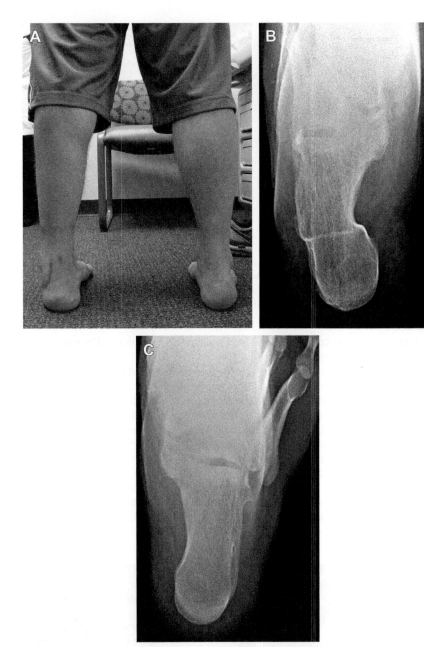

**Fig. 4.** Preoperative posterior clinical picture of a patient with an overcorrected flatfoot on the left (*A*). Bilateral axial radiographs showing moderate varus on the left (*B*), compared with normal right side (*C*).

osteotomy is performed (Dwyer), it is the author's preference to slightly superiorly translate the posterior tuberosity to lower the relative calcaneal pitch as described by Hansen (see **Fig. 5**G).[36] Some surgeon's prefer a Z-type osteotomy with a closing wedge that achieves more direct coronal plane correction.[31,32] In this procedure,

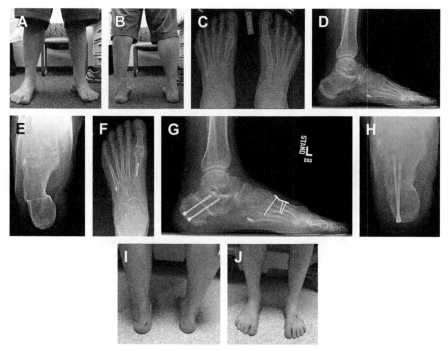

**Fig. 5.** Case example of an overcorrected flatfoot reconstruction treated surgically. Preoperative anterior and posterior clinical pictures (*A, B*). Preoperative anteroposterior (AP), lateral, and axial foot radiographs showing asymmetric talonavicular coverage, cavus foot deformity, and moderate varus hindfoot (*C–E*). Postoperative AP, lateral, and axial foot radiographs 4 months after revision lateralizing calcaneal osteotomy (Dwyer with slight superior translation), dorsiflexion first metatarsal osteotomy, and lateral ligament reconstruction (*F–H*). Postoperative anterior and posterior clinical pictures 7 months postoperative showing improved clinical alignment (*I, J*).

relative superior translation of the posterior tuberosity occurs as a result of the osteotomy (**Fig. 6**). However, it is the author's experience that more soft tissue dissection is required for this osteotomy and therefore care should be undertaken especially considering this is being performed through previously operated skin and soft tissue.

## LATERAL COLUMN LENGTHENING VERSUS CALCANEOCUBOID DISTRACTION ARTHRODESIS

To address significant foot abduction in AAFD, many surgeons use the lateral column lengthening (LCL) procedure. LCL is achieved through an osteotomy in the anterior process of the calcaneus or through a calcaneocuboid joint distraction arthrodesis.[6,7,18,19,37–41] Many surgeons prefer LCL through an osteotomy in the anterior process of the calcaneus because of the joint-preserving nature of this osteotomy and high reported rates of nonunion in calcaneocuboid distraction arthrodesis.[6,18,39] This is achieved multiple ways, most commonly through insertion of either autograft or allograft in the anterior process.[42,43] A Z-type LCL osteotomy has also been described.[32,44,45] While the LCL procedure can be very effective in correcting the abduction deformity, there may be residual forefoot supination deformity. In addition, too much lengthening can lead to an adducted midfoot position, which has been

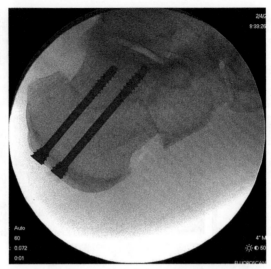

**Fig. 6.** Z-type calcaneal osteotomy with lateral-based closing wedge through the horizontal limb. Note the relative superior translation that occurs through the vertical limbs.

shown to lead to decreased patient outcomes in activities of daily living and quality of life.[46]

Lateral foot discomfort is one of the most common complaints after AAFD correction, and is often attributed to overlengthening of the lateral column (**Fig. 7**).[9,15,17–19,40] Clinically it is important to determine where exactly the patient is experiencing the lateral foot discomfort. Generalized lateral foot discomfort that is mostly plantar is likely related to overloading the lateral border of the foot while weight-bearing. Multiple studies have shown increases in lateral foot pressure after flatfoot

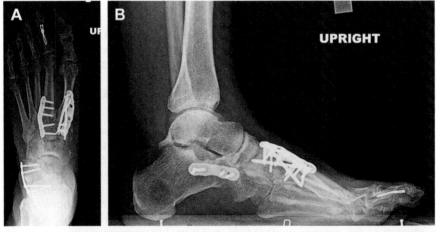

**Fig. 7.** Postoperative AP (*A*) and lateral (*B*) foot radiograph after flatfoot overcorrection via lateral column lengthening and first/second tarsometatarsal arthrodesis. Note the relative overcoverage of the talonavicular joint, plantarflexed first ray, and high calcaneal pitch creating a cavovarus foot alignment.

reconstructions, especially with LCL.[15,17,47–50] Cadaver studies have shown increased graft size correlates with increased plantar forefoot mean and peak pressure.[17] Fifth metatarsal stress fractures have also been reported (**Fig. 8**).[18,51] Alternatively, lengthening through the anterior process of the calcaneus can lead to increased contact pressure across the calcaneocuboid joint and resultant pain.[52] One cadaver study actually showed decreased calcaneocuboid joint pressure with LCL in comparison with a simulated flatfoot that was graft size dependent, but increased pressure compared with the intact foot.[53] Nonunion of either osteotomy or arthrodesis may also be a cause of lateral column pain (see **Fig. 3**B).[6,18,39,40]

Correcting an overlengthened lateral column is difficult. It is imperative to determine if there is residual forefoot supination. Technically, the lateral column may not be overlengthened as much as the medial column was undercorrected by not addressing the residual forefoot supination. This situation is addressed with a medial column procedure via dorsal opening wedge cuneiform (Cotton) osteotomy or a tarsometatarsal arthrodesis (see **Figs. 3** and **7**).[6,40,48,54–57] However, cadaver studies have shown conflicting data on whether lateral forefoot pressure changes after a Cotton osteotomy is added to LCL in a flatfoot reconstruction model.[48,49]

The overlengthened lateral column is shortened either through closing wedge osteotomy or shortening arthrodesis. Although shortening an overlengthened anterior process calcaneus is theoretically feasible, technically this is challenging. A lateral

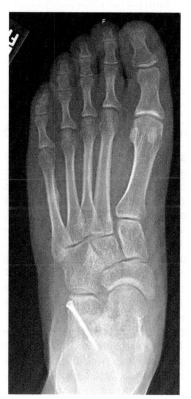

**Fig. 8.** Postoperative AP foot radiograph 8 months after lateral column lengthening with a healing fifth metatarsal stress fracture.

closing wedge osteotomy through the cuboid is performed, although it is more commonly described in pediatric conditions.[58] The closing wedge cuboid osteotomy is less powerful than a LCL through the anterior process and therefore full correction may be difficult to achieve. It is the author's opinion that shortening of the lateral column is best achieved through arthrodesis of the calcaneocuboid joint. Closing wedge osteotomy through a previously fused calcaneocuboid joint has also been described.[6] Standard joint preparation with removal of cartilage and subchondral bone may provide enough shortening; however, if more shortening is desired further bone resection can easily be performed. This procedure would also address any pain from increased pressure across this joint. Finally, a derotational cuboid osteotomy to correct the residual supination deformity of the foot has also been described in combination with triple arthrodesis.[59]

## MEDIAL COLUMN PROCEDURES

Addressing the medial column in flatfoot correction is often essential to achieve a plantigrade foot. Common reasons to require medial column intervention are residual supination of the forefoot after hindfoot correction is achieved and hypermobility with or without plantar gapping of the medial column joints (most commonly the first tarsometatarsal joint or the naviculocuneiform joint).[6,40,54,56,60] Arthrodesis is the preferred approach in the setting of hypermobility or degenerative changes in these joints.[6,40,60] Residual supination without hypermobility may be addressed with a dorsally based opening wedge medial cuneiform (Cotton) osteotomy (see **Fig. 3**).[54–57] Overcorrection of the medial column in combination with the other components of the flatfoot correction may lead to a plantarflexed first ray (see **Fig. 7**B). When this results in pain at the plantar first metatarsal head or sesamoids, surgical correction is considered. The most effective surgical treatment is a dorsiflexion closing wedge osteotomy through the base of the first metatarsal (see **Fig. 5**G). If the first tarsometatarsal (TMT) joint is arthritic or painful, a similar correction is performed through an arthrodesis of this joint with associated deformity correction (dorsal closing wedge or superior translation).

## ISOLATED HINDFOOT ARTHRODESIS VERSUS TRIPLE ARTHRODESIS

Patients with either a rigid AAFD or degenerative disease of the hindfoot joints often undergo hindfoot arthrodesis as part of the deformity correction. Which joint is fused depends on the clinical scenario. Isolated subtalar arthrodesis is an effective adjunct to previously mentioned flatfoot procedures.[61,62] With derotation and angulation of the subtalar joint, this arthrodesis may replace the need for a MDCO, LCL, or both.[62] Rigid AAFD is most commonly addressed with either triple arthrodesis or modified double arthrodesis (subtalar and talonavicular arthrodesis).[63–66] As in the joint-sparing techniques described previously, overcorrection during an arthrodesis procedure can occur, although undercorrection is again more common. Two technical errors can theoretically lead to overcorrection during an arthrodesis procedure. First, overpronation through the talonavicular or transverse tarsal joints can lead to increased pressure along the medial column and possible pain at the first metatarsal head. Similarly, overrotation through the subtalar joint, with possible varus positioning of the calcaneus in relation to the talus, can lead to varus hindfoot alignment (**Fig. 9**). In these circumstances, realignment osteotomies may need to be performed. The transverse tarsal joints are osteotomized and derotated into a plantigrade position.[59,67] The rotational deformity from an overrotated subtalar arthrodesis would likely have to be addressed through an osteotomy through the subtalar joint with deformity correction.[67] Alternatively, if the rotation is reasonable but there is residual hindfoot varus, a lateralizing

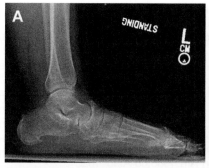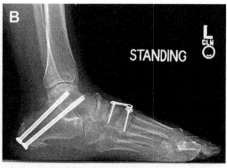

**Fig. 9.** Preoperative (*A*) and 3 months postoperative (*B*) lateral foot radiographs after flat-foot reconstruction including realignment subtalar arthrodesis and Cotton osteotomy. Note the relatively supinated forefoot despite using a plantarflexion osteotomy of the medial column through the medial cuneiform.

calcaneal osteotomy may be sufficient. Finally, a hindfoot arthrodesis that leads to a cavovarus foot can put significant stress on the lateral ankle ligaments, and/or pero-neal tendons. A lateral ligament reconstruction, peroneal tendon debridement or repair, or both may be required as part of the deformity correction if present.

## COMPLICATIONS

Similar to any revision surgery, surgically correcting an overcorrected flatfoot comes with inherent potential complications. Operating through previous incisions and resul-tant scar tissue can lead to wound healing problems and associated infections. This is particularly true on the lateral side of the hindfoot in the case of revising the MDCO, LCL, or subtalar arthrodesis. Nerve paresthesias are another common potential complication when operating through scar tissue. The sural nerve and its branches can be injured during revision osteotomies of the calcaneal tuberosity or anterior pro-cess of the calcaneus, in addition to calcaneocuboid arthrodesis.[6,9,18,43,68] The tibial nerve is at risk during lateralizing calcaneal osteotomy both from direct injury when performing the osteotomy and from compression secondary to the deformity correc-tion.[33–35] Finally, if full deformity correction is unable to be achieved with the previously described methods, residual foot deformity may lead to persistent symptoms.

## SUMMARY

The overcorrected flatfoot reconstruction is a complex problem that is challenging to treat. As with most orthopedic conditions, a thorough history and physical, including full evaluation of what was performed during the previous operation, is imperative to understand this clinical condition. Although symptoms often resemble those seen in a cavovarus foot, it is important to correlate the symptoms, physical examination find-ings, and imaging studies to determine the appropriate plan for treatment. Often sim-ple conservative treatments, such as offloading shoe inserts, orthotics, or bracing, may be enough to manage and control the patient's symptoms.

Operative intervention may be required in recalcitrant or more severe cases. The appropriate surgical procedure should be tailored to the patient's specific symptoms as it correlates with the portion of the previous operation that is deemed the cause of the overcorrection. Simple osteotomies of the calcaneus and/or first metatarsal may be sufficient. Alternatively, arthrodesis of one or multiple joints of the hindfoot and/or midfoot may be required to achieve a plantigrade foot. As always in these complex problems, combining soft tissue procedures, such as capsulotomies, tenolysis, or tendon lengthenings, may be needed as adjunct procedures for full correction.

## REFERENCES

1. Johnson KA, Strom DE. Tibialis posterior tendon dysfunction. Clin Orthop Relat Res 1989;239:196–206.
2. Mann RA, Thompson FM. Rupture of the posterior tibial tendon causing flatfoot. J Bone Joint Surg Am 1985;67-A:556–61.
3. Funk DA, Cass JR, Johnson KA. Acquired adult flat foot secondary to posterior tibial-tendon pathology. J Bone Joint Surg Am 1986;68-A:95–102.
4. Myerson MS. Adult acquired flatfoot deformity: treatment of dysfunction of the posterior tibial tendon. Instr Course Lect 1997;46:393–405.
5. Sangeorzan BJ, Mosca V, Hansen ST Jr. Effect of calcaneal lengthening on relationships among the hindfoot, midfoot, and forefoot. Foot Ankle 1993;14:136–41.
6. Toolan BC, Sangeorzan BJ, Hansen ST Jr. Complex reconstruction for the treatment of dorsolateral peritalar subluxation of the foot. Early results after distraction arthrodesis of the calcaneocuboid joint in conjunction with stabilization of, and transfer of the flexor digitorum longus tendon to, the midfoot to treat acquired pes planovalgus in adults. J Bone Joint Surg 1999;81-A:1545–60.
7. Moseir-Laclair S, Pomeroy G, Manoli A II. Intermediate follow-up on the double osteotomy and tendon transfer procedure for stage II posterior tibial tendon insufficiency. Foot Ankle Int 2001;22(4):283–91.
8. Hadfield MH, Snyder JW, Liacouras PC, et al. Effects of medializing calcaneal osteotomy on Achilles tendon lengthening and plantar foot pressures. Foot Ankle Int 2003;24:523–9.
9. Myerson MS, Badekas A, Schon LC. Treatment of stage II posterior tibial tendon deficiency with flexor digitorum longus tendon transfer and calcaneal osteotomy. Foot Ankle Int 2004;25(7):445–50.
10. Vora AM, Tien TR, Parks BG, et al. Correction of moderate and severe acquired flexible flatfoot with medializing calcaneal osteotomy and flexor digitorum longus transfer. J Bone Joint Surg Am 2006;88(8):1726–34.
11. Saltzman CL, el-Khoury GY. The hindfoot alignment view. Foot Ankle Int 1995; 16(9):572–6.
12. Yoshioka N, Ikoma K, Kido M, et al. Weight-bearing three-dimensional computed tomography analysis of the forefoot in patients with flatfoot deformity. J Orthop Sci 2016;21(2):154–8.
13. Deland JT. Adult-acquired flatfoot deformity. J Am Acad Orthop Surg 2008;16(7): 399–406.
14. Deland JT, Page A, Sung IH, et al. Posterior tibial tendon insufficiency results at different stages. HSS J 2006;2:157–60.
15. Ellis SJ, Yu JC, Johnson AH, et al. Plantar pressures in patients with and without lateral foot pain after lateral column lengthening. J Bone Joint Surg Am 2010; 92(1):81–91.
16. Iossi M, Johnson JE, McCormick JJ, et al. Short-term radiographic analysis of operative correction of adult acquired flatfoot deformity. Foot Ankle Int 2013; 34(6):781–91.
17. Oh I, Imhauser C, Choi D, et al. Sensitivity of plantar pressure and talonavicular alignment to lateral column lengthening in flatfoot reconstruction. J Bone Joint Surg Am 2013;95:1094–100.

18. Thomas RL, Wells BC, Garrison RL, et al. Preliminary results comparing two methods of lateral column lengthening. Foot Ankle Int 2001;22(2):107–19.
19. Kou JX, Balasubramaniam M, Kippe M, et al. Functional results of posterior tibial tendon reconstruction, calcaneal osteotomy, and gastrocnemius recession. Foot Ankle Int 2012;33(7):602–11.
20. Zaw H, Calder JDF. Operative management options for symptomatic flexible adult acquired flatfoot deformity: a review. Knee Surg Sports Traumatol Arthrosc 2010;18:135–42.
21. Hiller L, Pinney SJ. Surgical treatment of acquired flatfoot deformity: what is the state of practice among academic foot and ankle surgeons in 2002? Foot Ankle Int 2003;24:701–5.
22. Guyton GF, Jeng C, Krieger LE, et al. Flexor digitorurn longus transfer and medial displacement calcaneal osteotomy for posterior tibial tendon dysfunction: a middle-term clinical foiiow-up. Foot Ankle Int 2001;22(8):627–32.
23. Aronow MS. Tendon transfer options in managing the adult flexible flatfoot. Foot Ankle Clin 2012;17(2):205–26.
24. Takahashi M, Ward SR, Marchuk LL, et al. Asynchronous muscle and tendon adaptation after surgical tensioning procedures. J Bone Joint Surg Am 2010; 92(3):664–74.
25. Koutsogiannis E. Treatment of mobile flat foot by displacement osteotomy of the calcaneus. J Bone Joint Surg Br 1971;53(1):96–100.
26. Niki H, Hirano T, Okada H, et al. Outcome of medial displacement calcaneal osteotomy for correction of adult-acquired flatfoot. Foot Ankle Int 2012;33(11): 940–6.
27. Chan JY, Williams BR, Nair P, et al. The contribution of medializing calcaneal osteotomy on hindfoot alignment in the reconstruction of the stage II adult acquired flatfoot deformity. Foot Ankle Int 2013;34(2):159–66.
28. Conti MS, Ellis SJ, Chan JY, et al. Optimal position of the heel following reconstruction of the stage II adult-acquired flatfoot deformity. Foot Ankle Int 2015; 36(8):919–27.
29. Arangio GA, Salathe EP. A biomechanical analysis of posterior tibial tendon dysfunction, medial displacement calcaneal osteotomy and flexor digitorum longus transfer in adult acquired flat foot. Clin Biomech 2009;24(4):385–90.
30. Dwyer FC. Osteotomy of the calcaneum for pes cavus. J Bone Joint Surg Br 1959;41(1):80–6.
31. Malerba F, De Marchi F. Calcaneal osteotomies. Foot Ankle Clin 2005;10:523–40.
32. Scioli MW. Triple-step osteotomies of the calcaneus for the correction of varus and valgus deformities of the hindfoot. Tech Foot Ankle Surg 2009;8(1):10–6.
33. VanValkenburg S, Hsu RY, Palmer DS, et al. Neurologic deficit associated with lateralizing calcaneal osteotomy for cavovarus foot correction. Foot Ankle Int 2016; 37(10):1106–12.
34. Krause FG, Pohl MJ, Penner MJ, et al. Tibial nerve palsy associated with lateralizing calcaneal osteotomy: case reviews and technical tip. Foot Ankle Int 2009; 30(3):258–61.
35. Cody EA, Greditzer HG, MacMahon A, et al. Effects on the tarsal tunnel following malerba Z-type osteotomy compared to standard lateralizing calcaneal osteotomy. Foot Ankle Int 2016;37(9):1017–22.
36. Hansen ST. Osteotomy techniques. In: Hansen ST, editor. Functional reconstruction of the foot and ankle. Baltimore (MD): Lippincott Williams & Wilkins; 2000. p. 357–84.
37. Evans D. Calcaneo-valgus deformity. J Bone Joint Surg Br 1975;57(3):270–8.

38. Marks RM, Long JT, Ness ME, et al. Surgical reconstruction of posterior tibial tendon dysfunction: prospective comparison of flexor digitorum longus substitution combined with lateral column lengthening or medial displacement calcaneal osteotomy. Gait Posture 2009;29:17–22.

39. Grunander TR, Thordarson DB. Results of calcaneocuboid distraction arthrodesis. Foot Ankle Surg 2012;18:15–8.

40. Chi TD, Toolan BC, Sangeorzan BJ, et al. The lateral column lengthening and medial column stabilization procedures. Clin Orthop Relat Res 1999;365:81–90.

41. Chan JY, Greenfield ST, Soukup DS, et al. Contribution of lateral column lengthening to correction of forefoot abduction in stage IIb adult acquired flatfoot deformity reconstruction. Foot Ankle Int 2015;36(12):1400–11.

42. Dolan C, Henning J, Anderson J, et al. Randomized prospective study comparing tri-cortical iliac crest autograft to allograft in the lateral column lengthening component for operative correction of adult acquired flatfoot deformity. Foot Ankle Int 2007;28:8–12.

43. Grier KM, Walling AK. The use of tricortical autograft versus allograft in lateral column lengthening for adult acquired flatfoot deformity: an analysis of union rates and complications. Foot Ankle Int 2010;31(9):760–9.

44. Vander Griend R. Lateral column lengthening using a "Z" osteotomy of the calcaneus. Tech Foot Ankle Surg 2008;7(4):257–63.

45. Scott RT, Berlet GC. Calcaneal Z osteotomy for extra-articular correction of hindfoot valgus. J Foot Ankle Surg 2013;52(3):406–8.

46. Conti MS, Chan JY, Huong TD, et al. Correlation of postoperative midfoot position with outcome following reconstruction of the stage II adult acquired flatfoot deformity. Foot Ankle Int 2015;36(3):239–47.

47. Davitt JS, MacWilliams BA, Armstrong PF. Plantar pressure and radiographic changes after distal calcaneal lengthening in children and adolescents. J Pediatr Orthop 2001;21(1):70–5.

48. Benthien RA, Parks BG, Guyton GP, et al. Lateral column calcaneal lengthening, flexor digitorum longus transfer, and opening wedge medial cuneiform osteotomy for flexible flatfoot: a biomechanical study. Foot Ankle Int 2007;28(1):70–7.

49. Scott AT, Hendry TM, Iaquinto JM, et al. Plantar pressure analysis in cadaver feet after bony procedures commonly used in the treatment of stage II posterior tibial tendon insufficiency. Foot Ankle Int 2007;28(11):1143–53.

50. Tien TR, Parks BG, Guyton GP. Plantar pressures in the forefoot after lateral column lengthening: a cadaver study comparing the Evans osteotomy and calcaneocuboid fusion. Foot Ankle Int 2005;26(7):520–5.

51. Davitt JS, Morgan JM. Stress fracture of the fifth metatarsal after Evans' calcaneal osteotomy: a report of two cases. Foot Ankle Int 1998;19(10):710–2.

52. Cooper PS, Nowak MD, Shaer J. Calcaneocuboid joint pressures with lateral column lengthening (Evans) procedure. Foot Ankle Int 1997;18(4):199–205.

53. Xia J, Zhang P, Yang Y, et al. Biomechanical analysis of the calcaneocuboid joint pressure after sequential lengthening of the lateral column. Foot Ankle Int 2013;34(2):261–6.

54. Aiyer A, Dall GF, Shub J, et al. Radiographic correction following reconstruction of adult acquired flat foot deformity using the cotton medial cuneiform osteotomy. Foot Ankle Int 2016;37(5):508–13.

55. McCormick JJ, Johnson JE. Medial column procedures in the correction of adult acquired flatfoot deformity. Foot Ankle Clin 2012;17(2):283–98.

56. Hirose CB, Johnson JE. Plantarflexion opening wedge medial cuneiform osteotomy for correction of fixed forefoot varus associated with flatfoot deformity. Foot Ankle Int 2004;25(8):568–74.

57. Lutz M, Myerson M. Radiographic analysis of an opening wedge osteotomy of the medial cuneiform. Foot Ankle Int 2011;32(3):278–87.

58. Mubarak SJ, Van Valin SE. Osteotomies of the foot for cavus deformities in children. J Pediatr Orthop 2009;29(3):294–9.

59. Haddad SL. Surgical strategies: use of the cuboid osteotomy in combination with the triple arthrodesis with lateral column overload. Foot Ankle Int 2009;30(9): 904–11.

60. Ajis A, Geary N. Surgical technique, fusion rates, and planovalgus foot deformity correction with naviculocuneiform fusion. Foot Ankle Int 2014;35(3):232–7.

61. Johnson JE, Cohen BE, DiGiovanni BF, et al. Subtalar arthrodesis with flexor digitorum longus transfer and spring ligament repair for treatment of posterior tibial tendon insufficiency. Foot Ankle Int 2000;21(9):722–9.

62. Stephens HM, Walling AK, Solmen JD, et al. Subtalar repositional arthrodesis for adult acquired flatfoot. Clin Orthop Relat Res 1999;365:69–73.

63. Knupp M, Schuh R, Stufkens SA, et al. Subtalar and talonavicular arthrodesis through a single medial approach for the correction of severe planovalgus deformity. J Bone Joint Surg Br 2009;91:612–5.

64. Sammarco VJ, Magur EG, Sammarco GJ, et al. Arthrodesis of the subtalar and talonavicular joints for correction of symptomatic hindfoot malalignment. Foot Ankle Int 2006;27(9):661–6.

65. Schuh R, Salzberger F, Wanivenhaus AH, et al. Kinematic changes in patients with double arthrodesis of the hindfoot for realignment of planovalgus deformity. J Orthop Res 2013;31(4):517–24.

66. Ahmad J, Pedowitz D. Management of the rigid arthritic flatfoot in adults: triple arthrodesis. Foot Ankle Clin 2012;17(2):309–22.

67. Haddad SL, Myerson MS, Pell RF, et al. Clinical and radiographic outcome of revision surgery for failed triple arthrodesis. Foot Ankle Int 1997;18(8):489–99.

68. Silva MG, Tan SH, Chong HC, et al. Results of operative correction of grade IIB tibialis posterior tendon dysfunction. Foot Ankle Int 2015;36(2):165–71.

# The Undercorrected Flatfoot Reconstruction

Kenneth J. Hunt, MD[a],*, Ryan P. Farmer, MD[b]

## KEYWORDS

- Flatfoot undercorrection • Flatfoot malunion • Lateral column lengthening
- Medializing calcaneal osteotomy • Triple arthrodesis

## KEY POINTS

- Flatfoot deformities can be undercorrected in several planes.
- A clear understanding of the causes of flatfoot, and all components of the deformity, is critical to avoiding undercorrection.
- Strategies to rectify the symptomatic or biomechanically problematic, undercorrected flatfoot are outlined herein.

## INTRODUCTION

Adult flatfoot (or pes planovalgus) deformity is in most cases an acquired deformity. Though there are periods of developmental flatfoot during the toddler and adolescent stages of development, these typically resolve with continued growth and the concomitant decrease in ligamentous laxity.[1] Once skeletal maturity is achieved, loss of the medial longitudinal arch occurs in a combination of failure of static and dynamic structures, resulting in an inability of the hindfoot to lock during the gait cycle. Structural failure causes deformity at the midfoot joints, talonavicular joint, and tibiotarsal joints, leading to forefoot varus, midfoot abduction, and hindfoot valgus.[2] Each deformity must be addressed during surgical reconstruction to achieve appropriate correction and to mitigate the risk of recurrence or failure of the construct.

Though there are many causes of adult acquired flatfoot deformity (AAFD), most cases are associated with posterior tibialis tendon (PTT) dysfunction.[3] Most patients with symptomatic flatfoot develop failure of both static and dynamic supporting structures. Failure is typically brought on by ligamentous laxity, followed by dysfunction and subsequent insufficiency of the PTT.[2] Progressive laxity of the PTT, the primary

The authors have nothing to disclose.
[a] Foot and Ankle Surgery, Department of Orthopaedic Surgery, University of Colorado School of Medicine, 12631 East 17th Avenue, Room 4508, Aurora, CO 80045, USA; [b] Department of Orthopaedic Surgery, University of Colorado School of Medicine, 12631 East 17th Avenue, Room 4508, Aurora, CO 80045, USA
* Corresponding author.
*E-mail address:* kenneth.j.hunt@ucdenver.edu

Foot Ankle Clin N Am 22 (2017) 613–624
http://dx.doi.org/10.1016/j.fcl.2017.04.003
1083-7515/17/© 2017 Elsevier Inc. All rights reserved.

dynamic stabilizer of the medial longitudinal arch, then leads to failure of the spring ligament, resulting in progressive uncovering of the talar head and subsequent attenuation of the medial-sided joint capsules, and the long and short plantar ligaments. Ligamentous laxity is often found in the talocalcaneal interosseous ligament and, in more advanced disease, deltoid ligament insufficiency leads to ankle instability.[4] Regardless of cause or temporal considerations, a flatfoot deformity typically involves dorsolateral peritalar subluxation of the foot, and elongation, rupture, or failure of the medial soft tissue structures (eg, posterior tibial tendon, spring ligament, plantar ligaments, and joint capsules).

The number of osseous and soft tissue structures involved in a flatfoot deformity can make the approach to treatment complex. Bluman and colleagues[2] modification of the Johnson and Strom classification system is a helpful guide to surgical treatment. Although surgical treatments continue to evolve and long-term treatment outcomes are a major focus of current literature, there is a paucity of literature examining the impact of, and approach to, the treatment of the undercorrected flatfoot deformity. The focus of this article is to explore common undercorrections during surgical repair of a flatfoot deformity, including how these can be prevented and addressed. The underlying theme is that failure to restore both the bony architecture and the integrity of the medial soft tissue structures can put the patient at risk of recurrence due to persistent imbalance, which can lead to another failure of soft tissues, recurrence of bony deformity, and return of the pain and dysfunction that led to surgery to begin with.

## THE UNDERCORRECTED FLATFOOT

Undercorrection of a flatfoot is most often caused by failure to fully appreciate the extent of the deformity present or the underlying cause of the deformity, or failure to address each component adequately. For example, failing to recognize that the deformity is a rigid, rather than a flexible, deformity can be a component of undercorrection.[5] Treating a flexible deformity with soft tissue procedures alone will ultimately lead to failure of the procedure or recurrence of the deformity because the architecture of the foot, lax ligaments, and so forth have not been properly addressed. Failure to correct a rigid deformity may alter ambulatory mechanics such that other overstrained structures (typically on the medial side) might fail (**Fig. 1**).

In general, there are 3 deformities that need to be assessed during the preoperative evaluation and addressed intraoperatively if indicated: hindfoot valgus, midfoot abduction, and forefoot varus. This article explores the results of undercorrection of each of these deformities. The importance of soft tissues in these reconstructions cannot be underestimated, although failures of bony corrections are the more visible representations of undercorrection. The goal of restoring the bony anatomy is to first protect healing medial soft tissues and, ultimately, to restore normal ambulatory kinematics to prevent recurrence of deformity and symptoms. See later discussion of the appropriate surgical management options to address specific shortfalls in correction.

## CONSERVATIVE TREATMENTS

Before exploring surgical options, it is important to note that, in some cases of undercorrected flatfoot reconstruction, conservative management can alleviate or mitigate recurrence of symptoms, and perhaps slow progression of deformity. Such treatments include custom corrective orthoses, bracing, shoe modifications, strengthening of medial stabilizing structures, stretching of a tight triceps surae, and anti-inflammatory modalities. However, due to the potentially progressive nature of

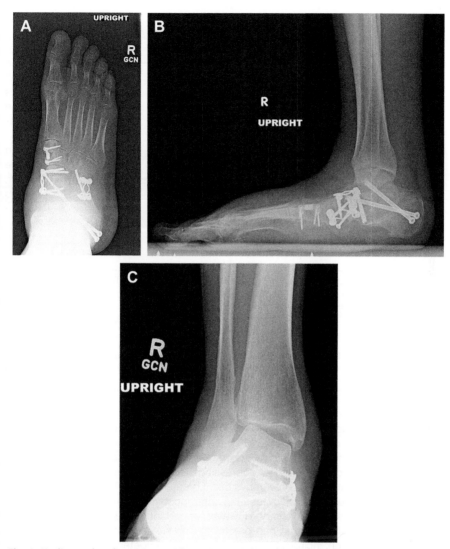

**Fig. 1.** Radiographs of a patient with previous triple arthrodesis and medial cuneiform dorsal opening wedge osteotomy (Cotton). (*A*) Oblique foot radiograph with healed fusion sites. (*B*) Lateral foot radiograph demonstrating collapse of the medial longitudinal arch and decreased talar-1st metatarsal angle. (*C*) Anteroposterior view (AP) of the ankle demonstrating ankle valgus with attenuation of the medial ligamentous structures.

recurrence, patients should be monitored closely and, if symptoms progress, surgical intervention to address the deformity should be undertaken (**Table 1**).[6–11]

### Correction of Hindfoot Valgus

Correction of hindfoot valgus by calcaneal osteotomy or subtalar arthrodesis is a standard component of surgical flatfoot correction. Restoration of hindfoot alignment is critical to prevent failure of the reconstruction, and to correct the abnormal gait

**Table 1**
**Description of surgical procedures for residual deformity**

| Deformity | Procedure | Indications | Contraindications |
|-----------|-----------|-------------|-------------------|
| Hindfoot valgus | Medializing calcaneal osteotomy | Flexible hindfoot valgus with <40% talar head uncovering | Rigid flatfoot, hindfoot arthritis[9] |
| | Subtalar arthroereisis | Subtalar eversion with hindfoot valgus | Subtalar arthritis, peroneal muscle spasm, excessive ligamentous laxity[6] |
| | Subtalar arthrodesis | Hindfoot valgus with subtalar arthrosis or degenerative changes | Compromised soft tissues or vascular dysfunction; correctable deformity[7] |
| Midfoot abduction | Calcaneal opening wedge osteotomy (Evans) | >40% talar head uncoverage, subfibular impingement[8] | Calcaneocuboid joint (CCJ) instability |
| | Calcaneocuboid distraction arthrodesis | Talar head undercoverage with CCJ arthrosis, degenerative changes or instability | None |
| Forefoot varus | Medial cuneiform dorsal opening wedge osteotomy | Forefoot varus or supination after hindfoot alignment with stable first tarsometatarsal (TMT) joint[10] | First TMT instability |
| | First TMT fusion | Persistent forefoot varus or supination with 1st TMT arthrosis/instability[10] | Nonarthritic, stable first TMT |

kinematics that can accompany hindfoot valgus.[12] The goal is to restore the anatomic alignment of 3° to 5° of valgus (**Fig. 2**).

The medializing calcaneal osteotomy is, in many cases, powerful enough to restore the medial longitudinal arch, even without addressing the lateral or medial column (**Fig. 3**).

The somewhat arbitrary rule of thumb is that if greater than 40% of the talar head is covered by the navicular on a weightbearing anteroposterior (AP) radiograph, a lateral column lengthening is not necessary. However, importantly, each patient is different and there are many factors that can predict the preservation of the reconstructed medial longitudinal arch, including tissue stiffness, the competence of the spring ligament, and the magnitude of the medial slide following the osteotomy. Failure to adequately shift the calcaneus can result in inadequate correction of both deformities, as evidenced by **Fig. 4**.

In addition to deformed bony architecture, attention must be paid to the role of the triceps surae and Achilles complex in the cause of flatfoot. Failure to properly identify and address a tight gastrocnemius or Achilles tendon as an exacerbating force in hindfoot deformity can lead to recurrence of hindfoot malposition or difficulty achieving intraoperative correction. With muscular imbalance and peritalar subluxation, a tight heel cord can transform the triceps surae from a primary heel inverter to a hindfoot evertor, causing further stress on the medial structures and resulting in further medial arch instability.[13,14] As further degenerative progression of the hindfoot valgus deformity occurs, Achilles tendon contracture becomes more apparent and must be recognized and addressed intraoperatively to avoid forefoot rotational dysfunction and lateral column overload. If the foot must be plantarflexed to passively correct the

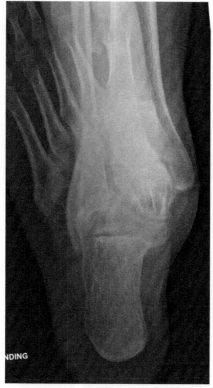

**Fig. 2.** Hindfoot alignment view demonstrating normal alignment of the heel relative to the shaft of the tibia.

hindfoot position, then a gastrocnemius recession or heel cord lengthening should be undertaken as part of flatfoot reconstruction[15] (**Fig. 5**). In addition, once the bony correction is achieved, adequate restoration of medial soft tissues is important to achieve long-term success. This includes, as indicated, PTT debridement, flexor digitorum longus (FDL) transfer to the navicular, and repair of the spring ligament.

### Correction of Midfoot Abduction

Weightbearing radiographs are an absolute necessity when evaluating flatfoot deformity. Evaluation of talar head undercoverage by the navicular on an AP radiograph will provide an indication of the amount of midfoot abduction that is present. As previously alluded to, talar head uncovering of greater than 40% should prompt consideration of a procedure to lengthen the lateral column of the foot and to treat the deformity present at the transverse tarsal joint. Lateral column lengthening procedures largely consist of the calcaneal opening wedge osteotomy and calcaneocuboid distraction arthrodesis. The authors prefer lateral column lengthening through a calcaneus anterior process opening wedge osteotomy with corticocancellous graft (**Fig. 6**).

Although there is controversy surrounding the appropriate indications of the 2 procedures, multiple studies have noted increased complications with calcaneocuboid distraction arthrodesis and equivalent patient satisfaction results.[16,17] Though it has been demonstrated that an anterior calcaneus osteotomy can increase

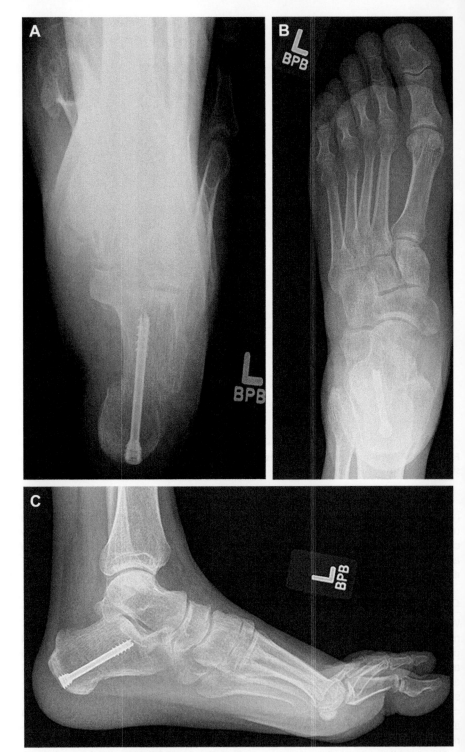

**Fig. 3.** Postoperative radiographs of a patient who underwent flatfoot reconstruction with medial displacement calcaneal osteotomy (MIDCO) alone. (*A*) Hindfoot alignment view after medializing calcaneal slide osteotomy with improvement of the medial distal tibial angle. (*B*) AP of the foot with appropriate talar head coverage and well positioned calcaneus. (*C*) Lateral of the foot with preservation of the medial arch.

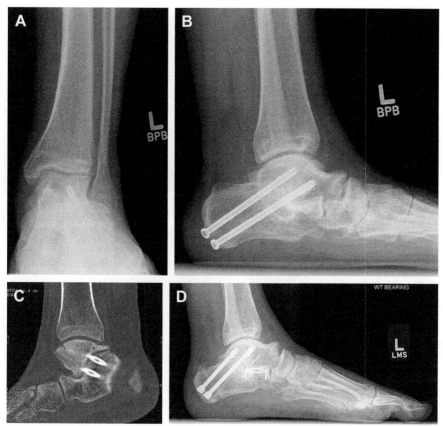

**Fig. 4.** Radiographs of a patient with persistent lateral ankle pain, nonunion, and malunion following subtalar arthrodesis for flatfoot deformity. (*A*) AP of the ankle demonstrating calcaneofibular impingement. (*B*) Lateral ankle radiograph demonstrating loss of the medial arch and decreased calcaneal pitch angle and talus-first metatarsal angle. (*C*) Sagittal computed tomography image demonstrating nonunion of subtalar fusion. (*D*) Postoperative lateral radiograph following revision surgery, including revision subtalar fusion, MDCO, and lateral column lengthening.

calcaneocuboid joint (CCJ) pressures there is no definitive evidence that this leads to joint degeneration.[18]

Failure to address the lateral column in the presence of an abducted forefoot can lead to recurrence or failure of the construct due to excessive stresses on the medial soft tissues. If this is identified, the appropriate treatment is to perform an adequate lateral column lengthening to restore normal mechanics. Although it can be difficult to judge intraoperatively, the amount of correction achieved with lateral column lengthening is key to successful outcomes. Overcorrection with lateral column lengthening can result in substantially increased loads on the lateral column.[19] (See Todd A. Irwin's article, "Overcorrected Flatfoot Reconstruction," in this issue).

### Correction of Forefoot Position

Following correction of hindfoot valgus and midfoot abduction, assessment of forefoot supination or varus must be evaluated due to rigidity of the forefoot with persistent

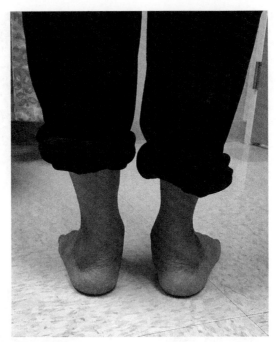

**Fig. 5.** Clinical photograph of a patient with pes planovalgus deformity with severe hind-foot valgus and collapse of the medial arch with demonstration of the too many toes sign.

supination leading to increased pressure in the lateral forefoot and subsequent over-load.[20] Though many procedures exist for medial column stabilization, the authors recommend the use of either a first tarsometatarsal (TMT) arthrodesis or medial cune-iform opening wedge osteotomy (Cotton osteotomy[21]). Evaluation of the stability of

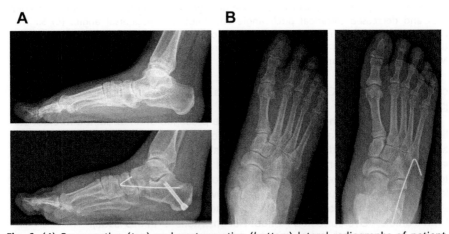

**Fig. 6.** (A) Preoperative (top) and postoperative (bottom) lateral radiographs of patient treated with medializing calcaneal osteotomy and lateral column lengthening through calcaneal anterior process opening wedge osteotomy. (B) Preoperative (left) and postoper-ative (right) AP radiographs demonstrating improved forefoot abduction and improved coverage of the talar head by the navicular.

the first TMT joint will assist in making the surgical decision between the 2 procedures. Consideration of the lateral weightbearing radiograph can demonstrate plantar surface first TMT joint gapping, indicating joint instability. Presence of first TMT joint instability or arthritis is an indication to pursue first TMT arthrodesis rather than a medial cuneiform osteotomy.[2]

## PERIOPERATIVE CONSIDERATIONS

When preparing to address an undercorrected flatfoot, as with any revision surgery, evaluation of the soft tissues and overall patient health assessment should be performed. Evaluation of failed surgeries should also include routine blood work that includes C-reactive protein, erythrocyte sedimentation rate, and complete blood count to assess for infectious sources of failure. Following an appropriate workup, additional information should be obtained from the patient and include the previous operative report whenever possible. Advanced imaging may also be necessary to evaluate for fusion of previous joint arthrodesis. Following full formal evaluation, surgical intervention should include a stepwise approach to the patient with undercorrected flatfoot. This should be undertaken to ensure that all persistent deformities are identified and addressed (**Fig. 7**). The modified Johnson-Strom classification system[22] introduced by Bluman and colleagues[2] provides a road-map for this evaluation. A careful physical and radiographic examination with weightbearing images can facilitate understanding of residual deformity and further surgical intervention can then be planned. After the completion of any further surgical correction, the remaining deformity should be evaluated and further procedures considered. In general, correction should be conducted in a hindfoot to forefoot manner with forefoot supination or varus corrected last. The outcomes following surgical treatments are summarized in **Table 2**.[5,9,15–17,23–28]

## COMPLICATIONS AND MANAGEMENT

This article is generally directed toward the management of undercorrection following previous flatfoot surgery, which is in and of itself a complication. Persistent

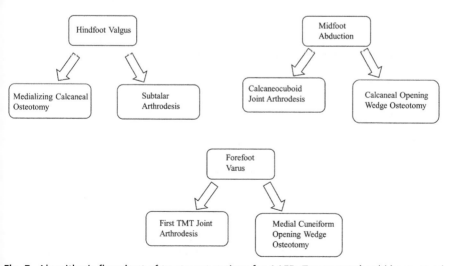

**Fig. 7.** Algorithmic flowchart of treatment options for AAFD. Treatment should be pursued beginning with hindfoot correction, followed by evaluation and correction of midfoot abduction, with forefoot supination evaluated after correction of the midfoot and hindfoot.

**Table 2**
**Clinical outcomes of surgical corrections of flatfoot deformity**

| Deformity | Procedure | Outcomes |
|---|---|---|
| Hindfoot valgus | Achilles tendon lengthening | Used in conjunction with medializing calcaneal osteotomy (MCO) and FDL transfer excellent results obtained[14] |
| | MCO | 92% satisfaction at mean 5-y follow-up[9] |
| | Subtalar arthroereisis | Improved American Orthopedic Foot and Ankle Society (AOFAS) scores in 40 subjects in 2 studies at 15 and 44-mo follow-up[22,23] |
| | Subtalar arthrodesis | Near 100% rate of fusion with solitary arthrodesis[24] |
| Midfoot abduction | Calcaneal opening wedge osteotomy (Evans) | Equivocal AOFAS scores, fewer complications than CCJ arthrodesis[15,16] |
| | Calcaneocuboid distraction arthrodesis | Increased nonunion and complication rate[5,25] |
| Forefoot varus | Medial cuneiform dorsal opening wedge osteotomy | Lutz and Myerson[8] noted significant improvement in forefoot radiographic parameters in 110 subjects |
| | First TMT fusion | >90% union rate in multiple studies[26] |

undercorrection is a continued complication of further flatfoot surgical intervention. In general, nonunion and malunion are complications of any osteotomy with different rates based on the type of procedure performed, graft usage, and surgical technique:

- Medializing calcaneal osteotomy: rare nonunion complication with at least 50% bony contact and up to 10 to 15 mm translation. Medial-sided soft tissues are at risk during breach of the medial cortex. Forefoot abduction cannot be corrected without additional procedures.[29]
- Subtalar arthrodesis: favorable to excellent outcomes with favorable to high patient satisfaction as measured by the AOFAS with follow-up from 15 months to 9 years. Fusion rate was greater than 86% with hardware removal from 13% to 22% of cases.[30]
- Calcaneal opening wedge osteotomy (Evans): can increase pressure within the CCJ, resulting in degenerative joint changes, though rate of progression to osteoarthritis is unknown.[6]
- CCJ arthrodesis: increased complication rate compared with Evans procedure, with increased rates of nonunion and delayed union.[17] There are increased plantar pressures under the fifth metatarsal head compared with Evans.[7]
- Medial cuneiform opening wedge osteotomy (Cotton): largest presented series with 10% complication rate from symptomatic hardware, lateral column overload, and deformity recurrence.[8]
- First TMT arthrodesis: nonunion rates range from 4% to 12%, possibly related to surgical technique.[27,28]

## POSTOPERATIVE CARE

Depending on the amount of surgical intervention required and the presence or absence of bony procedures, postoperative immobilization will consist of 2 weeks in a plaster splint followed by a period of nonweightbearing in either a short leg cast or stiff postoperative boot. With stable osteotomies, the authors' preference is nonweightbearing in a boot from 2 to 6 weeks postoperative so that soft tissue swelling can be addressed and joints can be mobilized. For fusion procedures, we favor a cast from 2 to 6 weeks postoperative to facilitate fusion. At 6 weeks, weightbearing radiographs are obtained to confirm bone healing and maintenance of corrected foot position. Weightbearing begins at 6 weeks and formal physical therapy to restore strength, balance, and proprioception (and normal gait) is undertaken.

## SUMMARY

Revision surgery for the undercorrected flatfoot is similar to the primary surgery given that the deformity and driving forces must be understood and a comprehensive surgical treatment plan formulated. Formal evaluation should include advanced imaging, as necessary, to evaluate for bony fusion of previous osteotomy sites and, if necessary, to evaluate the deformity. The revision surgeon must also consider soft tissue deficiencies and scar formation. Following a stepwise plan of corrective action and evaluating the foot position after each procedure will help to avoid undercorrection in the future.

## REFERENCES

1. Pfeiffer M, Kotz R, Ledl T, et al. Prevalence of flat foot in preschool-aged children. Pediatrics 2006;118(2):634–9.
2. Bluman EM, Title CI, Myerson MS. Posterior tibial tendon rupture: a refined classification system. Foot Ankle Clin 2007;12(2):233–49, v.
3. Beals TC, Pomeroy GC, Manoli A 2nd. Posterior tibial tendon insufficiency: diagnosis and treatment. J Am Acad Orthop Surg 1999;7(2):112–8.
4. Vulcano E, Deland JT, Ellis SJ. Approach and treatment of the adult acquired flatfoot deformity. Curr Rev Musculoskelet Med 2013;6(4):294–303.
5. Lin JS, Myerson MS. The management of complications following the treatment of flatfoot deformity. Instr Course Lect 2011;60:321–34.
6. Roche AJ, Calder JD. Lateral column lengthening osteotomies. Foot Ankle Clin 2012;17(2):259–70.
7. Tien TR, Parks BG, Guyton GP. Plantar pressures in the forefoot after lateral column lengthening: a cadaver study comparing the Evans osteotomy and calcaneocuboid fusion. Foot Ankle Int 2005;26(7):520–5.
8. Lutz M, Myerson M. Radiographic analysis of an opening wedge osteotomy of the medial cuneiform. Foot Ankle Int 2011;32(3):278–87.
9. Myerson MS, Badekas A, Schon LC. Treatment of stage II posterior tibial tendon deficiency with flexor digitorum longus tendon transfer and calcaneal osteotomy. Foot Ankle Int 2004;25(7):445–50.
10. Needleman RL. A surgical approach for flexible flatfeet in adults including a subtalar arthroereisis with the MBA sinus tarsi implant. Foot Ankle Int 2006;27(1): 9–18.
11. Guyton GP, Jeng C, Krieger LE, et al. Flexor digitorum longus transfer and medial displacement calcaneal osteotomy for posterior tibial tendon dysfunction: a middle-term clinical follow-up. Foot Ankle Int 2001;22(8):627–32.
12. Svoboda Z, Honzikova L, Janura M, et al. Kinematic gait analysis in children with valgus deformity of the hindfoot. Acta Bioeng Biomech 2014;16(3):89–93.
13. Myerson MS. Adult acquired flatfoot deformity: treatment of dysfunction of the posterior tibial tendon. Instr Course Lect 1997;46:393–405.
14. Trnka HJ, Easley ME, Myerson MS. The role of calcaneal osteotomies for correction of adult flatfoot. Clin orthopaedics Relat Res 1999;365:50–64.

15. Neufeld SK, Myerson MS. Complications of surgical treatments for adult flatfoot deformities. Foot Ankle Clin 2001;6(1):179–91.
16. Haeseker GA, Mureau MA, Faber FW. Lateral column lengthening for acquired adult flatfoot deformity caused by posterior tibial tendon dysfunction stage II: a retrospective comparison of calcaneus osteotomy with calcaneocuboid distraction arthrodesis. J Foot Ankle Surg 2010;49(4):380–4.
17. Thomas RL, Wells BC, Garrison RL, et al. Preliminary results comparing two methods of lateral column lengthening. Foot Ankle Int 2001;22(2):107–19.
18. Iaquinto JM, Wayne JS. Effects of surgical correction for the treatment of adult acquired flatfoot deformity: a computational investigation. J Orthop Res 2011;29(7):1047–54.
19. Oh I, Imhauser C, Choi D, et al. Sensitivity of plantar pressure and talonavicular alignment to lateral column lengthening in flatfoot reconstruction. J Bone Joint Surg Am 2013;95(12):1094–100.
20. Benthien RA, Parks BG, Guyton GP, et al. Lateral column calcaneal lengthening, flexor digitorum longus transfer, and opening wedge medial cuneiform osteotomy for flexible flatfoot: a biomechanical study. Foot Ankle Int 2007;28(1):70–7.
21. Cotton FJ. Foot Statics and Surgery. New England Journal of Medicine 1936;214(8):353–62.
22. Johnson KA, Strom DE. Tibialis posterior tendon dysfunction. Clin orthopaedics Relat Res 1989;239:196–206.
23. Zhu Y, Xu XY. Treatment of stage II adult acquired flatfoot deformity with subtalar Arthroereises. Foot Ankle Spec 2015;8(3):194–202.
24. Ozan F, Dogar F, Gencer K, et al. Symptomatic flexible flatfoot in adults: subtalar arthroereisis. Ther Clin Risk Manag 2015;11:1597–602.
25. Kitaoka HB, Patzer GL. Subtalar arthrodesis for posterior tibial tendon dysfunction and pes planus. Clin Orthop Relat Res 1997;(345):187–94.
26. Toolan BC, Sangeorzan BJ, Hansen ST Jr. Complex reconstruction for the treatment of dorsolateral peritalar subluxation of the foot. Early results after distraction arthrodesis of the calcaneocuboid joint in conjunction with stabilization of, and transfer of the flexor digitorum longus tendon to, the midfoot to treat acquired pes planovalgus in adults. J Bone Joint Surg Am 1999;81(11):1545–60.
27. McCormick JJ, Johnson JE. Medial column procedures in the correction of adult acquired flatfoot deformity. Foot Ankle Clin 2012;17(2):283–98.
28. Thompson IM, Bohay DR, Anderson JG. Fusion rate of first tarsometatarsal arthrodesis in the modified Lapidus procedure and flatfoot reconstruction. Foot Ankle Int 2005;26(9):698–703.
29. Guha AR, Perera AM. Calcaneal osteotomy in the treatment of adult acquired flatfoot deformity. Foot Ankle Clin 2012;17(2):247–58.
30. Diezi C, Favre P, Vienne P. Primary isolated subtalar arthrodesis: outcome after 2 to 5 years followup. Foot Ankle Int 2008;29(12):1195–202.

# Management of the Malunited Triple Arthrodesis

Jeffrey D. Seybold, MD

## KEYWORDS

• Triple arthrodesis • Malunion • Revision • Osteotomy

## KEY POINTS

- The best method to address a malunited triple arthrodesis is to avoid malunion in the first place; careful attention to the biomechanics of the foot and preoperative planning are critical, particularly when approaching a revision scenario.
- Standing evaluation and radiographic analysis identify the primary deformities: valgus or varus hindfoot, midfoot and forefoot supination or pronation, midfoot and forefoot abduction or adduction, and rocker bottom deformity.
- A stepwise and systematic approach to deformity correction is recommended, progressing from proximal to distal.
- Multiplanar deformity is common and must be addressed with a combination of osteotomies or resecting biplanar wedges of bone from the previous transverse tarsal arthrodesis site.
- Few clinical data are available, although available studies demonstrate excellent patient satisfaction and good correction of deformity after revision procedures.

## INTRODUCTION

Triple arthrodesis is a "time honored and effective technique of stabilizing and correcting painful hindfoot deformities"[1] and is frequently used in the treatment of a flatfoot deformity in the presence of subtalar and transverse tarsal arthritis, severe hindfoot rigidity, or in older and low-demand patients. Success rates for the procedure generally range above 85% throughout the literature, with most patients reporting they would undergo the procedure again if presented with the same treatment options.[2–9] The converse of these results could be read, however, as failure rates of the procedure approaching 15%. Nonunion is the most common complication reported after triple arthrodesis, with rates ranging in the literature from 10% to 23%,[2,4,8,10–12] although

Disclosure: The author is a paid consultant for Acumed and MedShape and serves on the editorial advisory board for *Foot and Ankle Clinics*.
Twin Cities Orthopedics, 4010 West 65th Street, Edina, MN 55435, USA
*E-mail address:* jseybold@tcomn.com

Foot Ankle Clin N Am 22 (2017) 625–636
http://dx.doi.org/10.1016/j.fcl.2017.04.009
foot.theclinics.com

improved hardware design and use of biologic stimulation have led to greater than 95% successful arthrodesis rates in recent years.[3,5–7,9,10] Although nonunion rates have decreased, the rates of deformity recurrence or of undercorrection or overcorrection of deformity have not changed dramatically and remain a source of procedure failure and patient dissatisfaction. Rates of malunion after triple arthrodesis are reported as high as 6% in the literature, with equinovarus with or without a rocker bottom deformity the most common position of malunion.[3,10,13] Even after revision triple arthrodesis, malunion is reported in as many as 7% of patients and recurrence of deformity in 3.5%.[13] Although numerous studies have evaluated the techniques and results of triple arthrodesis, few have evaluated strategies for addressing the malunited triple arthrodesis.[10,13–15] The focus of this article is to review the available literature regarding the malunited triple arthrodesis and present a treatment algorithm to address residual deformity.

## PATIENT EVALUATION

Although the point may seem intuitive, it bears stating that the best method to address a malunited hindfoot arthrodesis is to avoid malunion in the first place. In general, comprehensive understanding of the biomechanics of the hindfoot, careful preoperative planning, and meticulous execution of the index arthrodesis procedure limit the risk of malunion. Careful attention must be paid to soft tissue balancing around the ankle and hindfoot during the index procedure, and lengthening of the Achilles or gastrocnemius is often performed to limit residual pull on the posterior calcaneus by the Achilles complex into valgus. A tenotomy of the peroneal tendons may also be helpful in the spastic flatfoot deformity to allow for adequate correction of the valgus hindfoot. Inability to recognize and address residual forefoot supination after correction of the chronic flatfoot deformity leads to recurrence of hindfoot deformity as the forefoot attempts to remain plantigrade. Overcorrection of a flatfoot deformity is poorly tolerated and best avoided by reducing and stabilizing the talonavicular joint prior to the subtalar joint when correcting the hindfoot. Lateral overload and pain under the calcaneocuboid joint can be avoided if plantar subluxation of the cuboid is identified and corrected prior to arthrodesis of the calcaneocuboid joint. Techniques to identify and avoid these pitfalls have been discussed at length throughout this issue and are not the focus of this review.

Once the hindfoot is fused in a malunited position, soft tissue balancing alone is not sufficient to address the deformity. A careful patient examination is critical to assess the alignment of the fusion mass, the effect on the ankle joint, and any residual or compensatory midfoot or forefoot deformity. Standing evaluation reveals any gross malalignment of the hindfoot or asymmetry. Callus buildup may be noted over areas of prominent bone as a result of persistent deformity, particularly under the plantar foot or along the lateral column. A patient's prior surgical incisions should be noted, because further operative intervention may require an altered approach to avoid skin or soft tissue necrosis, especially in the setting of severe hindfoot valgus when closure of the lateral hindfoot incisions may prove difficult.

Radiographic evaluation is critical to identify the apex and degree of residual deformity present. Standing radiographs of the foot and ankle are typically required, and axial calcaneus or Saltzman hindfoot views are often helpful to provide a measurement of the varus or valgus of the hindfoot present and assist with preoperative planning. The advent of weight-bearing CT imaging has presented a useful tool for surgeons, providing a more detailed evaluation of the deformity present as well as assessing for adequate healing across the arthrodesis sites.

## OPERATIVE TECHNIQUES

A systematic approach to the correction of the malunited triple arthrodesis is critical to ensure that every aspect of the deformity is adequately addressed. Haddad and colleagues[13] presented a treatment algorithm in their patient series that remains a helpful guide and tackles deformity in a proximal to distal method to achieve adequate correction. Bibbo and colleagues[10] provided similar recommendations to address hindfoot deformity. Stephens and Saleh[14] and Toolan[15] presented small patient series using a single hindfoot osteotomy with satisfactory results. Although adequate correction of deformity was noted in these studies, the technical challenges in performing a single osteotomy for multiplanar deformity correction and limited cohort size in these series lend caution to enthusiastically endorsing these approaches without further study.

### Hindfoot Valgus

Although undercorrection of a flatfoot deformity is generally better tolerated than overcorrection into varus, persistent hindfoot valgus may lead to continued subfibular impingement pain, fibular stress fractures, deltoid ligament strain, and valgus load on the ankle, leading to deformity and arthritis. Typically, a medial displacement calcaneal osteotomy is sufficient to address the residual hindfoot valgus.[10,13] An oblique incision is made over the posterior calcaneal tuberosity plantar to the peroneal tendon sheath, avoiding injury to the sural nerve. The periosteum overlying the calcaneal tuberosity is elevated. Hohmann retractors are placed around the dorsal and plantar aspects of the tuberosity and an oscillating saw is used to complete the osteotomy. The preoperative hindfoot alignment view may provide a guide for the amount of translation required to adequately correct the deformity, but typically at least 8 mm to 10 mm of medial translation is required. The osteotomy is commonly secured with a single compression screw inserted in percutaneous fashion through the posterior heel, although multiple compression plate or staple implants are available and may limit the potential risk of prominent hardware. Medial closing or lateral opening wedge osteotomies are not necessary to address this deformity. Patients are immobilized in a short leg splint for 2 weeks postoperatively and transition to a tall cast boot. Weight-bearing activity is allowed in the boot at 6 weeks postoperatively and patients may then transition to a comfortable shoe as tolerated.

### Hindfoot Varus

Although encountering an isolated varus hindfoot malunion without concomitant forefoot or midfoot deformity is uncommon, this deformity can be corrected with a lateral displacement closing wedge osteotomy of the calcaneal tuberosity (**Fig. 1**).[10,13] The approach to the lateral calcaneus is described previously, and 2 saw cuts are created, taking care to create the apex of the closing wedge at the medial cortex of the calcaneus. Care must be taken in this scenario not to overtranslate the posterior tuber because the shift of the bone laterally decreases volume within the tarsal tunnel and may lead to an iatrogenic tarsal tunnel syndrome.[16,17] Postoperative care proceeds in a similar manner to the medial displacement calcaneal osteotomy, as described previously. A closing wedge osteotomy alone without translation of the posterior tuber may not be sufficient to adequately correct the varus malalignment, as demonstrated in a cadaver study evaluating a closing wedge Z-osteotomy of the calcaneus.[18]

For more severe deformity or deformity associated with midfoot or forefoot supination or pronation deformity, correction may be achieved through either a lateral

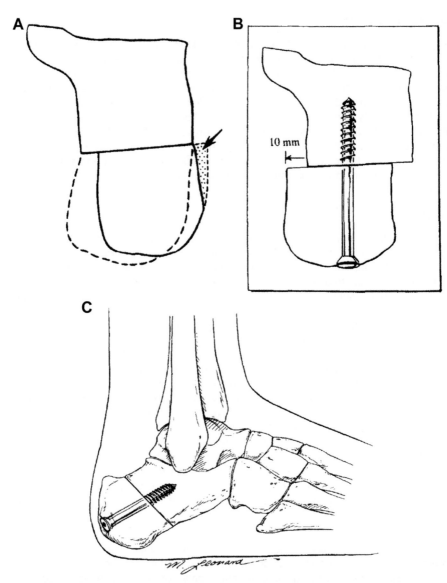

**Fig. 1.** Varus deformity of the hindfoot may be addressed by both removing a closing wedge from the lateral aspect of the calcaneus (*A*), and translating the posterior tuberosity laterally (*B*). The osteotomy is commonly secured with a single screw inserted through the posterior heel (*C*). (*From* Haddad SL, Myerson MS, Pell RF 4th, et al. Clinical and radiographic outcome of revision surgery for failed triple arthrodesis. Foot Ankle Int 1997;18(8):492; with permission.)

displacement calcaneal osteotomy or a closing wedge osteotomy at the level of the subtalar joint, in conjunction with a rotational osteotomy through the transverse tarsal joints (**Figs. 2** and **3**). The transverse tarsal osteotomy must be performed if removing a wedge from the subtalar joint; otherwise, the subtalar joint osteotomy does not close down.[13]

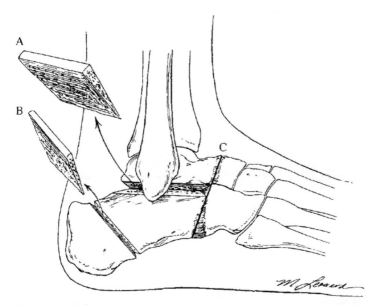

**Fig. 2.** When varus deformity is more severe and associated with excessive supination through the midfoot and forefoot, a combination of osteotomies is required. A closing wedge osteotomy through the subtalar joint (*A*) is a powerful alternative to an osteotomy through the calcaneal tuberosity (*B*), but must communicate with the transverse tarsal osteotomy (*C*) otherwise the subtalar joint osteotomy will not close down. (*From* Haddad SL, Myerson MS, Pell RF 4th, et al. Clinical and radiographic outcome of revision surgery for failed triple arthrodesis. Foot Ankle Int 1997;18(8):491; with permission.)

*Forefoot Supination or Pronation*

A derotational osteotomy is required to address persistent supination or pronation deformity of the midfoot and forefoot (**Fig. 4**).[4,7] Two incisions are used: the medial incision is placed in the interval between the anterior and posterior tibialis tendons; the lateral incision starts along a standard sinus tarsi approach but deviates more plantarward to end near the fifth tarsometatarsal joint. Soft tissue dissection is carried down to bone through both incisions at the level of the prior transverse tarsal joints and soft tissue retractors are placed around the dorsal and plantar foot. An oscillating saw is used to complete an osteotomy across the transverse tarsal arthrodesis and the foot is rotated into a plantigrade position. A combination of compression screws, staples, and compression plates may be used to secure the osteotomy medially and laterally. Care should be taken to preserve enough navicular and cuboid bone distal to the osteotomy to accommodate adequate fixation of the hardware.

*Forefoot Abduction or Adduction*

A closing wedge osteotomy through the transverse tarsal joint is used to correct coronal plane malalignment of the forefoot (**Fig. 5**).[6] A similar approach to the transverse tarsal joints is used, as described previously. Kirschner wires inserted under fluoroscopic guidance may be helpful to ensure the osteotomy saw cuts are made along the appropriate planes. An osteotomy is created perpendicular to the plane of the hindfoot. A second osteotomy is then created perpendicular to the plane of the forefoot. A medial closing wedge is completed for forefoot abduction and a lateral closing wedge is created for forefoot adduction. Once the osteotomy is closed down, a

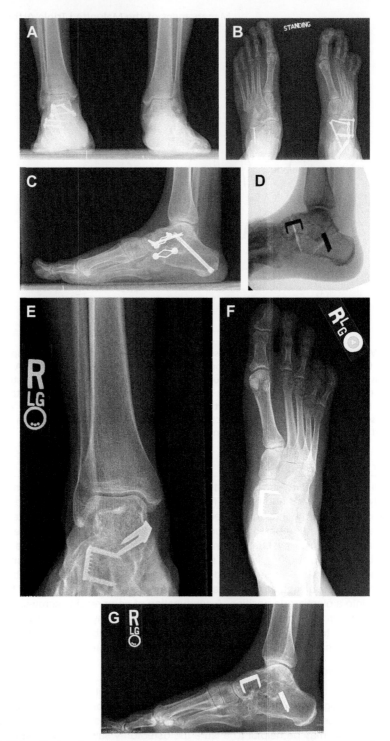

**Fig. 3.** This patient underwent a prior triple arthrodesis with residual hindfoot varus and midfoot supination deformity (*A-C*), as can be seen particularly on the weight-bearing foot radiographs (*B*). A lateral closing wedge and translational osteotomy of the calcaneus was performed in addition to a derotational osteotomy through the transverse tarsal fusion mass (*D*). Postoperative radiographs demonstrate improved alignment of the hindfoot with a plantigrade first ray (*E-G*).

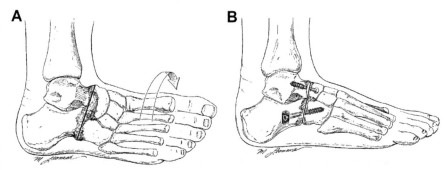

**Fig. 4.** Excessive midfoot and forefoot supination or pronation can be addressed through a derotational osteotomy performed through the prior transverse tarsal fusion mass (*A*). Care should be taken to leave enough bone distally at the navicular and cuboid to allow for adequate fixation (*B*) (*From* Haddad SL, Myerson MS, Pell RF 4th, et al. Clinical and radiographic outcome of revision surgery for failed triple arthrodesis. Foot Ankle Int 1997;18(8):493; with permission.)

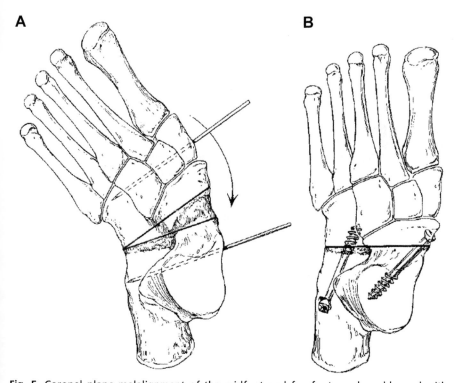

**Fig. 5.** Coronal plane malalignment of the midfoot and forefoot can be addressed with either a medially based or laterally based closing wedge osteotomy through the prior transverse tarsal fusion mass (*A*). Again, care should be taken to leave enough bone distally at the navicular and cuboid to allow for adequate fixation (*B*) (*From* Haddad SL, Myerson MS, Pell RF 4th, et al. Clinical and radiographic outcome of revision surgery for failed triple arthrodesis. Foot Ankle Int 1997;18(8):493; with permission.)

combination of compression screws, staples, and compression plates is used to secure the osteotomy. Care should be taken again to preserve enough navicular and cuboid bone distal to the osteotomy to accommodate adequate fixation of the hardware. The initial postoperative protocol follows the same restrictions as the calcaneal osteotomy but weight bearing is typically advanced slowly at the 6-week mark, with full weight bearing typically achieved in a boot by 9 weeks to 10 weeks postoperatively. Patients wean from a protective boot to a shoe at 12 weeks postoperatively. Opening wedge osteotomies are typically avoided in this scenario because bone graft is required and increases the number of bone surfaces to heal. In addition, overlengthening of the hindfoot and midfoot may lead to excessive tension on surrounding neurovascular structures with subsequent paresthesias or vascular compromise distally in the toes and lesser toe deformities as a result of a tenodesis effect.[10]

### Rocker Bottom Deformity

The rocker bottom deformity is present typically from a malunited calcaneocuboid joint, because the cuboid subluxes plantarly after the talonavicular and subtalar joints have been reduced during the index triple arthrodesis. A uniplanar deformity may be corrected with a plantar closing wedge osteotomy through the transverse tarsal joints (**Fig. 6**).[13] The exposure is completed, as described previously for the transverse tarsal osteotomy, and the prominent plantar bone is removed through the resected plantar wedge.

### Combination Deformities

It is unusual to encounter the deformities, discussed previously, in an isolated fashion. By using the principles behind each of these osteotomies, biplanar wedges of bone may be removed from the transverse tarsal joint to address any combination of these deformities (**Fig. 7**). In these scenarios, the deformity should be approached from proximal to distal, with the hindfoot malalignment addressed first, followed by any midfoot or forefoot malrotation or angulation. Guide wires are frequently helpful in this situation and are advanced across the hindfoot along the planned osteotomy cuts to ensure adequate and appropriately placed wedges of bone are removed.

**A**          **B**

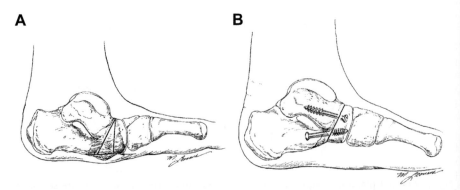

**Fig. 6.** A plantar wedge of bone can be removed from the transverse tarsal joint fusion mass to address persistent rocker bottom deformity (*A*). Care must be taken to leave sufficient distal bone to allow for fixation of the osteotomy (*B*). (*From* Haddad SL, Myerson MS, Pell RF 4th, et al. Clinical and radiographic outcome of revision surgery for failed triple arthrodesis. Foot Ankle Int 1997;18(8):494; with permission.)

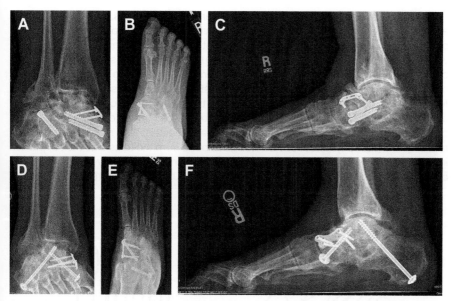

**Fig. 7.** This patient presented with persistent ankle and lateral hindfoot pain after a prior triple arthrodesis complicated by a subtalar nonunion (the patient had also already had subtalar screws removed). Clinically, the patient demonstrated severe residual hindfoot valgus with nearly 30 of excessive abduction of the midfoot and a rocker bottom deformity (*A-C*). The patient underwent revision subtalar arthrodesis performed with medial translation of the calcaneus to correct the hindfoot valgus, and a medially based and plantarly based closing wedge osteotomy through the transverse tarsal fusion mass to address the abduction and rocker bottom deformity. An anterior ankle cheilectomy was also performed to address the significant anterior joint line bony impingement (*D-F*). The patient was very satisfied with the position of the foot postoperatively with near complete relief of pain.

## RESULTS

Few case series have been published that review the results of revision triple arthrodesis, and the studies available present a limited number of patients. Haddad and colleagues[13] presented the results of revision triple arthrodesis in 28 patients (29 feet) with an average follow-up of 4.4 years (range 2–7 years). Patients with neuropathic arthropathy were excluded, and a majority of index procedures were performed for posttraumatic or rheumatoid arthritis or deformity. Two patients presented initially with posterior tibial tendon insufficiency. Multiplanar deformity of the triple arthrodesis was the most frequently encountered (10 feet), with 8 varus deformities, 5 valgus deformities, and 2 rocker bottom deformities. Average time to a revision arthrodesis was 3.7 years from the index procedure, and patients underwent an average of 3 prior foot procedures after the initial triple arthrodesis before undergoing intervention with the investigators. Average time to bone healing was reported as 8.9 weeks. All patients would undergo the procedure again and radiographic measures of correction all improved (although not statistically significant). Seventeen feet did not require a custom shoe or orthotic postoperatively. Four patients (14%) reported major complications, which required further operative intervention although 7 actual major complications were noted, including malunion or recurrent deformity or a wound problem requiring surgical intervention. Seven patients reported minor complications, bringing the total number of patients with complications to 11 (39%).

The malunited triple arthrodesis with persistent hindfoot valgus, forefoot abduction, and rocker bottom deformity is addressed with a medial displacement calcaneal osteotomy and biplanar transverse tarsal osteotomy with a medial and plantar closing wedge using the algorithm, discussed previously. Toolan[15] described an opening-closing wedge osteotomy through the transverse tarsal joints to address this deformity, limiting need for a separate calcaneal osteotomy and preserving length of the foot (**Fig. 8**). The apex of the distal limb of the transverse tarsal osteotomy was truncated at the lateral talar head/neck, wedging open the lateral column as the medial column was compressed. A biplanar wedge was resected, with more bone resected medially and plantarly. The resected wedge of bone from the talus was then impacted into the lateral opening wedge upside-down. This single osteotomy achieved significant improvement in all clinical and radiographic outcome measures at an average

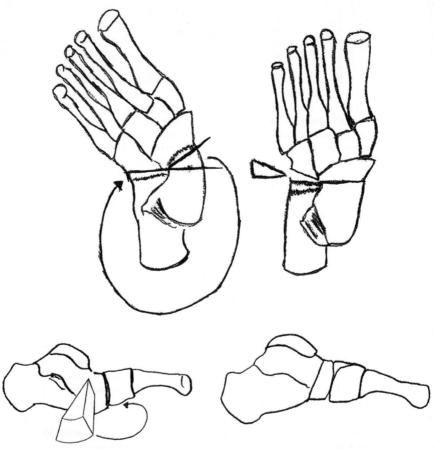

**Fig. 8.** One alternative to using a combination of osteotomies to address multiplanar deformity is the opening-closing wedge osteotomy described by Toolan. The apex of the transverse tarsal osteotomy is truncated at the lateral talar head/neck (*upper left*), wedging open the lateral column as the medial column is compressed (*upper right*). A medially based and plantarly based wedge is resected and then impacted into the lateral opening upside-down (*lower images*). (*From* Toolan BC. Revision of failed triple arthrodesis with an opening-closing wedge osteotomy of the midfoot. Foot Ankle Int 2004;25(7):457; with permission.)

of 18 months postoperatively (range 13–32 months). No major complications were reported and all patients were satisfied with the procedure. One superficial wound infection was noted and 1 patient underwent a subsequent procedure to remove hardware and a painful bony prominence along the opening wedge. Concerns regarding this study include a small sample size (5 patients) and the use of an opening wedge osteotomy, which increases the potential for nonunion if the implanted wedge does not fit adequately.

The first series to report results for revision triple arthrodesis was presented by Stephens and Saleh in 1994.[14] A single crescentic osteotomy was created through the hindfoot with satisfactory results reported in 5 patients. Although adequate correction of either equinovarus (4 patients) or hindfoot valgus (1 patient) deformity was reported, the investigators did not comment on the effect of this osteotomy on persistent or residual midfoot or forefoot deformity. In addition, the technical challenges performing this osteotomy, including creating concentric surfaces of bone and avoiding wound healing issues with the distal curl of the surgical incision in the setting of a previous sinus tarsi incision, would limit enthusiasm for this approach without further study.

## SUMMARY

Malunion after triple arthrodesis is one of the most common complications of the procedure and can present significant problems for patients and orthopedic surgeons. Revision procedures that realign the hindfoot and forefoot have been met with good success in limited reports. A systematic approach to creating osteotomies that correct residual or recurrent deformity is critical to achieving adequate correction and patient satisfaction. A step-by-step approach, correcting deformity from proximal to distal, ensures that all aspects of the deformity are addressed and a plantigrade foot is achieved. Further studies are warranted to adequately evaluate the success and failures of the various procedures, described previously.

## ACKNOWLEDGMENTS

The author would like to thank Dr J. Chris Coetzee and Dr Jacob Zide for their invaluable insight to this difficult clinical problem and assistance providing patient images.

## REFERENCES

1. Bennett GL, Graham CE, Mauldin DM. Triple arthrodesis in adults. Foot Ankle 1991;12(3):138–43.
2. Angus PD, Cowell HR. Triple arthrodesis. A critical long-term review. J Bone Joint Surg Br 1986;68(2):260–5.
3. Bednarz PA, Monroe MT, Manoli A 2nd. Triple arthrodesis in adults using rigid internal fixation: an assessment of outcome. Foot Ankle Int 1999;20(6):356–63.
4. Graves SC, Mann RA, Graves KO. Triple arthrodesis in older adults. Results after long-term follow-up. J Bone Joint Surg Am 1993;75(3):355–62.
5. Knupp M, Skoog A, Tornkvist H, et al. Triple arthrodesis in rheumatoid arthritis. Foot Ankle Int 2008;29(3):293–7.
6. Pell RF 4th, Myerson MS, Schon LC. Clinical outcome after primary triple arthrodesis. J Bone Joint Surg Am 2000;82(1):47–57.
7. Rosenfeld PF, Budgen SA, Saxby TS. Triple arthrodesis: is bone grafting necessary? The results in 100 consecutive cases. J Bone Joint Surg Br 2005;87(2): 175–8.

8. Saltzman CL, Fehrle MJ, Cooper RR, et al. Triple arthrodesis: twenty-five and forty-four-year average follow-up of the same patients. J Bone Joint Surg Am 1999;81(10):1391–402.
9. Sangeorzan BJ, Smith D, Veith R, et al. Triple arthrodesis using internal fixation in treatment of adult foot disorders. Clin orthop Relat Res 1993;(294):299–307.
10. Bibbo C, Anderson RB, Davis WH. Complications of midfoot and hindfoot arthrodesis. Clin Orthop Relat Res 2001;(391):45–58.
11. Friedenberg ZB. Arthrodesis of the tarsal bones; a study of failure of fusions. Arch Surg 1948;57(1):162–70.
12. Wilson FC Jr, Fay GF, Lamotte P, et al. Triple arthrodesis. a study of the factors affecting fusion after three hundred and one procedures. J Bone Joint Surg Am 1965;47:340–8.
13. Haddad SL, Myerson MS, Pell RF 4th, et al. Clinical and radiographic outcome of revision surgery for failed triple arthrodesis. Foot Ankle Int 1997;18(8):489–99.
14. Stephens M, Saleh J. Calcaneal dome osteotomy: a new procedure for revising triple arthrodesis. Foot Ankle Int 1994;15(7):368–71.
15. Toolan BC. Revision of failed triple arthrodesis with an opening-closing wedge osteotomy of the midfoot. Foot Ankle Int 2004;25(7):456–61.
16. Bruce BG, Bariteau JT, Evangelista PE, et al. The effect of medial and lateral calcaneal osteotomies on the tarsal tunnel. Foot Ankle Int 2014;35(4):383–8.
17. Cody EA, Greditzer HG 4th, MacMahon A, et al. Effects on the tarsal tunnel following malerba z-type osteotomy compared to standard lateralizing calcaneal osteotomy. Foot Ankle Int 2016;37(9):1017–22.
18. Zanolli DH, Glisson RR, Utturkar GM, et al. Calcaneal "Z" osteotomy effect on hindfoot varus after triple arthrodesis in a cadaver model. Foot Ankle Int 2014; 35(12):1350–7.

# Severe Stage 2: Fuse or Reconstruct

Scott B. Shawen, MD[a],*, Theodora C. Dworak, MD[b]

## KEYWORDS

- Stage II posterior tibial tendon dysfunction • Acquired flat foot deformity • Fusion
- Reconstruction

## KEY POINTS

- Surgical treatment of stage II posterior tibial tendon dysfunction is highly variable and depends on patient age, level of function, severity of deformity, and neurologic involvement.
- Flat foot reconstruction with joint and motion preservation is traditionally indicated for young patients with flexible deformity and no adjacent joint osteoarthritis.
- Triple arthrodesis of the subtalar, calcaneal cuboid, and the talonavicular joints, or double arthrodesis of the subtalar and talonavicular joints, is indicated in older patients with lower demand and/or chronic osteoarthritic change in the affected joints, or in patients with a neurologic origin of the flatfoot deformity.

## INTRODUCTION

Stage II posterior tibial tendon dysfunction or adult acquired flat foot deformity can be difficult to treat with a single surgical approach. Patients who meet the requirements for stage II disease can have a myriad of deformity and symptoms; therefore, surgical intervention must be tailored to the patient's specific condition. The severity of the deformity, patient functional level, age, comorbidities, and potential underlying neurologic cause must be considered to determine the best course of treatment. This article examines when fusion, verses reconstruction, is the appropriate treatment of patients with severe stage II posterior tibial tendon dysfunction.

## CLASSIFICATION

Posterior tibial tendon dysfunction or adult acquired flat foot deformity was first described by Johnson and Strom[1] in 1989 and was originally classified into 3 stages. Patients with stage I disease exhibit pain along the posterior tibial tendon and have

The author has nothing to disclose.
[a] OrthoCarolina Foot & Ankle Institute, 250 N Caswell Road #200, Charlotte, NC 28207, USA;
[b] Walter Reed National Military Medical Center, 8900 Wisconsin Avenue, Bethesda, MD 20889, USA
* Corresponding author.
E-mail address: scott.b.shawen@gmail.com

mild weakness with single-limb heel rise but have minimal deformity. As the condition progresses to stage II, patients develop increasing difficulty with the single-limb heel rise and display severe weakness of the posterior tibial tendon due to elongation and degeneration of the tendon.[1,2] As a result, the hind foot begins to develop a valgus position, but this deformity remains flexible. In stage III disease, the position of the hindfoot remains fixed in valgus. A fourth stage, added by Myerson[3] in 1997, is characterized by the deformity expanding to the ankle joint, with the talus also falling into valgus, and the development of osteoarthritic changes in the ankle. These stages are helpful to guide treatment; however, stage II affects a large group of patients with a spectrum of disease severity; therefore, treatment within this category can vary.

Due to the complexity of posterior tibial tendon dysfunction and help guide surgical treatment, in 2007, Bluman and colleagues[4] expanded the classification system to consider not only the position of the hind foot but also deformity of the forefoot and medial column instability. Patients with stage IIA1 have flexible forefoot varus in addition to flexible hind foot valgus, whereas patients with stage IIA2 have fixed forefoot varus. Stage IIB patients exhibit forefoot abduction in addition to flexible hind foot varus and stage IIIC patients have medial column instability, fixed forefoot varus, and continue to have flexible hind foot valgus.[4] This expansion of the classification system stratified patients who were previously considered to have similar disease manifestation.

## PATIENT EVALUATION

The treatment of any foot and ankle condition should begin with through history and physical examination. Patients who are early in the disease process often report medial ankle pain and swelling, due to tendinopathy, along the posterior tibial tendon.[5] Medial ankle pain can dissipate as patients progress in deformity and disease process. Additionally, careful attention to physical examination findings should focus on the presence of the too many toes sign, and the ability of the patient to do a single-limb heel rise on the affected extremity.[3] Physical examination of the hind foot to determine if the valgus deformity is fixed or flexible will separate stage II patients who are likely to benefit from reconstruction from stage III patients who will require triple arthrodesis.[6]

Radiologic evaluation with weightbearing views of the ankle and foot are used to evaluate talar-first metatarsal angle, calcaneal pitch, and lateral column height.[7] Degenerative changes in the subtalar, talonavicular, and calcaneal cuboid joints should also be noted because severe osteoarthritic changes at these joints may preclude reconstructive options.[8] Hind foot alignment views show the position of the calcaneus relative to the tibia but maybe difficult to interpret consistently.[9]

The position of the forefoot and hind foot can be challenging to determine in patients with severe flat foot deformity. Computerized tomography (CT) scans have traditionally been used to further characterize the 3-dimensional relationship of foot and ankle. However, in patients with flexible flat foot deformity, a traditional nonweightbearing CT scan may underestimate deformity. Recently, weightbearing CT scans have become increasingly available and can provided a more accurate representation of a patient's deformity during weightbearing.[10,11] MRI for flat foot evaluation is not traditionally needed; however, it can provide information about the condition of the posterior tibial tendon and flexor digitorum longus tendon, which may help determine surgical treatment.[12]

## RECONSTRUCTION

Stage II posterior tibial tendon dysfunction has traditionally been treated with reconstruction with favorable results in young patients. Deland[5] retrospectively reviewed the American Orthopedic Foot and Ankle Society Score (AOFAS) hind foot and the Short Form Health Survey (SF)-36 score in patients younger than the age of 50 years who underwent reconstruction for stage II posterior tibial tendon dysfunction. The mean increase in AOFAS score was 29.5 and the average physical function component of the SF-36 was 79.2.[13] Soukup and colleagues[14] demonstrated that obese subjects with stage II posterior tibial tendon dysfunction who undergo flat foot reconstruction have similar outcomes to normal weight subjects despite having worse symptoms, pain scores, and increased comorbidities before surgery. Similarly, Myerson and colleagues[15] described their results of stage II posterior tibial tendon dysfunction treated with flexor digitorum longus transfer and medial slide calcaneal osteotomy in 129 subjects. Only 4 subjects reported they were dissatisfied with their outcome, 125 subjects (93%) experienced pain relief, and 121 subjects had improvement in their

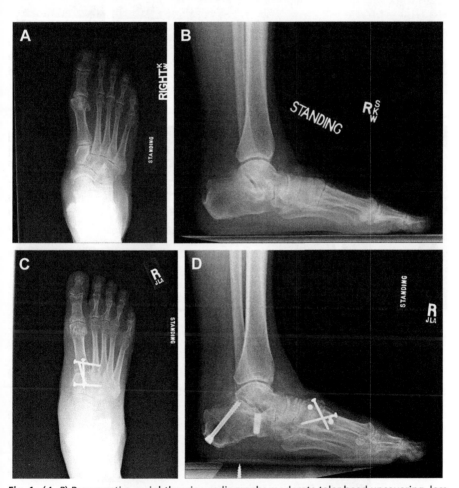

**Fig. 1.** (*A, B*) Preoperative weightbearing radiographs moderate talar head uncovering, loss of calcaneal pitch, and a break in the Meary line at the talonavicular joint. (*C, D*) Postoperative weightbearing radiographs after medial displacement calcaneal osteotomy, lateral column lengthening, Lapidus fusion, and soft tissue procedures, including a gastrocnemius recession, posterior tibial tendon debridement, and flexor digitorum longus tendon transfer.

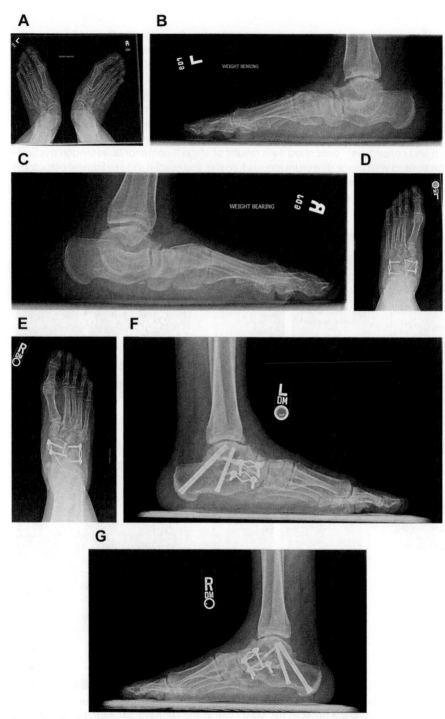

**Fig. 2.** (*A–C*) Preoperative weightbearing radiographs demonstrating severe pes planus with minimal talar head uncovering, severe forefoot abduction deformity, and loss of calcaneal pitch. (*D–G*) Postoperative weightbearing radiographs with near-normal alignment on the anteroposterior and lateral views. Residual talar osteophytes are present, as is common with this severity of deformity.

functional outcome scores. Reconstruction remains a good surgical option in the appropriate patient with stage II disease.

## CASE DISCUSSION
*Case 1*

A middle-aged female with a history of long-term pes planus with progressive posterior medial ankle pain without history of trauma was treated with casting and controlled ankle motion (CAM) walker with temporary benefit. Examination demonstrated hind foot valgus, inability to perform a single-limb heel rise, contracted Achilles, forefoot abduction, and fixed forefoot varus (**Fig. 1A, B**). She was treated with gastrocnemius recession, medial displacement calcaneal osteotomy, calcaneal lateral column lengthening (Evans), posterior tibial tendon debridement, flexor digitorum longus tendon transfer, and Lapidus fusion of the first tarsometatarsal (TMT) joint (see **Fig. 1C, D**).

## FUSION

There is a subset of patients with severe stage II posterior tibial tendon dysfunction that may benefit from hind foot fusion rather than reconstruction. Most often, these patients are older with comorbidities and have lower demand or have a neurologic origin to the deformity. Patients with osteoarthritis of the talar navicular joint or subtalar joint may benefit from a primary fusion because flat foot reconstruction techniques are unlikely to resolve patient's osteoarthritic pain. Additionally, patients with neuropathic deformity or decreased sensation secondary to peripheral neuropathy should be treated with fusion in contrast to reconstruction. Flat foot reconstruction in this patient population is likely to break down due to patients' lack of protective sensation.

Although patients who receive triple arthrodesis for flat foot reconstruction have traditionally had stage III disease, they continue to have favorable outcomes. Bednarz and colleagues[16] described their results of 57 subjects who received triple arthrodesis for a variety of foot conditions and showed a significant increase in AOFAS hind foot scores with minimal complications. Röhm and colleagues[17] described their outcomes of modified triple arthrodesis through a single medial incision in 84 subjects for flat foot deformity. At-5 year follow-up, no subject had loss of correction, mean AOFAS score was 67, and the visual analog scale score was 2.4.

## CASE DISCUSSION
*Case 2*

An active-duty Navy corpsman with progressive pain and difficulty with running began active duty in the Navy 4 years before presentation. Examination demonstrated a supple and correctable foot with severe hind foot valgus, forefoot abduction, fixed forefoot varus, and tight Achilles (**Fig. 2A–C**). He was treated with staged bilateral gastrocnemius recession and triple arthrodesis with lateral column lengthening through the calcaneal cuboid joint (see **Fig. 2 D–G**).

## SUMMARY

Stage II posterior tibial tendon dysfunction is a complex condition with varying clinical presentations. Careful evaluation with history, physical examination, and imaging must be synthesized to establish appropriate treatment of each patient. Younger, more active patients without significant adjacent degenerative joint disease may benefit from flat foot reconstruction. However, older patients with less physical demand and advanced degenerative changes, patients with more severe flexible pes planus, and patients with an underlying neurologic condition are likely to have a more reliable outcome with a double or triple arthrodesis.

## REFERENCES

1. Johnson KA, Strom DE. Tibialis posterior tendon dysfunction. Clin Orthop Relat Res 1989;(239):196–206.
2. Gonçalves-Neto J, Witzel SS, Teodoro WR, et al. Changes in collagen matrix composition in human posterior tibial tendon dysfunction. Joint Bone Spine 2002;69(2):189–94.
3. Myerson MS. Adult acquired flatfoot deformity: treatment of dysfunction of the posterior tibial tendon. Instr Course Lect 1997;46:393–405.
4. Bluman EM, Title CI, Myerson MS. Posterior tibial tendon rupture: a refined classification system. Foot Ankle Clin 2007;12(2):233–49, v.
5. Deland JT. Adult-acquired flatfoot deformity. J Am Acad Orthop Surg 2008;16(7): 399–406.
6. Abousayed MM, Tartaglione JP, Rosenbaum AJ, et al. Classifications in brief: Johnson and Strom classification of adult-acquired flatfoot deformity. Clin Orthop Relat Res 2016;474(2):588–93.
7. Younger AS, Sawatzky B, Dryden P. Radiographic assessment of adult flatfoot. Foot Ankle Int 2005;26(10):820–5.
8. Coughlin MJ, Saltzman CL, Anderson RB. Mann's surgery of the foot and ankle. Philadelphia: Saunders; 2014.
9. Sensiba PR, Coffey MJ, Williams NE, et al. Inter-and intraobserver reliability in the radiographic evaluation of adult flatfoot deformity. Foot Ankle Int 2010;31(2): 141–5.
10. Hirschmann A, Pfirrmann CWA, Klammer G, et al. Upright cone CT of the hindfoot: comparison of the non-weight-bearing with the upright weight-bearing position. Eur Radiol 2014;24(3):553–8.
11. Yoshioka N, Ikoma K, Kido M, et al. Weight-bearing three-dimensional computed tomography analysis of the forefoot in patients with flatfoot deformity. J Orthop Sci 2016;21(2):154–8.
12. Khoury NJ, El-Khoury GY, Saltzman CL, et al. MR imaging of posterior tibial tendon dysfunction. AJR Am J Roentgenol 1996;167(3):675–82.
13. Tellisi N, Lobo M, O'Malley M, et al. Functional outcome after surgical reconstruction of posterior tibial tendon insufficiency in patients under 50 years. Foot Ankle Int 2008;29(12):1179–83.
14. Soukup DS, MacMahon A, Burket JC, et al. Effect of obesity on clinical and radiographic outcomes following reconstruction of stage II adult acquired flatfoot deformity. Foot Ankle Int 2016;37(3):245–54.
15. Myerson MS, Badekas A, Schon LC. Treatment of stage II posterior tibial tendon deficiency with flexor digitorum longus tendon transfer and calcaneal osteotomy. Foot Ankle Int 2004;25(7):445–50.
16. Bednarz PA, Monroe MT, Manoli A 2nd. Triple arthrodesis in adults using rigid internal fixation: an assessment of outcome. Foot Ankle Int 1999;20(6):356–63.
17. Röhm J, Zwicky L, Lang TH, et al. Mid-to long-term outcome of 96 corrective hindfoot fusions in 84 patients with rigid flatfoot deformity. Bone Joint J 2015; 97-B(5):668–74.

# Pediatric Flatfoot
## Pearls and Pitfalls

Samuel E. Ford, MD, Brian P. Scannell, MD*

## KEYWORDS

- Pediatric • Pes planus • Flatfoot • Hindfoot valgus • Orthoses • Evans procedure
- Calcaneal lengthening osteotomy • Calcaneal-cuboid-cuneiform osteotomy

## KEY POINTS

- Asymptomatic, flexible flatfoot is a normal childhood variant that decreases in prevalence as children reach preteenage years.
- Conservative measures in the initial management of symptomatic flatfoot include Achilles stretching and both prefabricated and custom in-shoe orthoses.
- The calcaneal lengthening osteotomy (Evans procedure) and calcaneal-cuboid-cuneiform osteotomy are both surgical options for children with overall good outcomes.
- Arthrodesis is associated with long-term adjacent joint arthritis, including the tibiotalar joint; thus, the procedure is not routinely recommended for use in children and is considered a salvage procedure by most surgeons for ambulatory patients.
- Surgical treatment outcomes of painful flexible flatfeet are reported to be good to excellent in most (85%–95%) patients. Long-term follow-up studies are still needed.

## INTRODUCTION

Many children have physiologic flatfeet, which is almost uniformly asymptomatic and flexible. When flatfeet become painful and/or stiff, there is often a role for orthopedic involvement in the patient's care. A full differential must be explored via a complete patient evaluation, including history, physical examination, and imaging studies, before intervention may be recommended. There is little evidence that nonoperative measures, including medications, physical therapy, and orthoses/braces, are effective in addressing symptoms or deformity. Operative options include hindfoot/midfoot osteotomies, arthroereisis, and arthrodesis, different procedures have varying profiles of efficacy, long-term outcomes, and complications. Most procedural options have strong outcome profiles that relieve patients of their symptoms and correct associated deformities.

Disclosures: The authors have nothing to disclose.
Department of Orthopaedic Surgery, Levine Children's Hospital, Carolinas HealthCare System, 1025 Morehead Medical Drive, Suite 300, Charlotte, NC 28204, USA
* Corresponding author.
E-mail address: brian.scannell@carolinashealthcare.org

Foot Ankle Clin N Am 22 (2017) 643–656
http://dx.doi.org/10.1016/j.fcl.2017.04.008
1083-7515/17/© 2017 Elsevier Inc. All rights reserved.
foot.theclinics.com

In order for surgeons to advise parents, it is critical that they understand the normal variation encountered among childhood feet. Infants are commonly born with flatfeet, and the longitudinal arch forms over the first decade of life. Among children 3 to 6 years of age, 44% have flatfeet with an average 5.5° of hindfoot valgus. From age 3 to 6, the prevalence of flatfeet decreases from 54% to 24% as the arch matures.[1] Boys' arches mature in a delayed fashion relative to girls', 1 year later. Flatfeet tend to persist among overweight and obese children.[1,2]

The flatfoot deformity has been defined as a complex, variable deformity, which includes excessive plantarflexion of the talus, subtalar eversion during weight bearing, and a combination of valgus, external rotation, and dorsiflexion of the calcaneus relative to the talar head.[1,3] The navicular also becomes abducted and dorsiflexed relative to the talar head, drawing the entire midfoot and forefoot into abduction and supination relative to the hindfoot. These deformities result in a "shortened" lateral column, as first described by Evans in 1975, although it is not clear whether this is a true length discrepancy or functional difference due to talonavicular joint malalignment.[4] In addition, an Achilles contracture can develop, plantarflexing the hindfoot and driving stresses through the talonavicular joint during the midstance phase of gait through the underlying soft tissues.[3]

Types of flatfeet typically seen in children and adolescents include the following:

- Flexible flatfeet
- Flexible flatfoot with Achilles tightness
- Rigid flatfoot
  - Coalition (talocalcaneal, calcaneonavicular)
  - Congenital vertical talus
  - Skewfoot
  - Neurogenic flatfoot (eg, myelomeningocele, cerebral palsy, poliomyelitis)

## PATIENT EVALUATION OVERVIEW
### History

It is important to approach the history of these patients as follows in order to help to differentiate physiologic from pathologic flatfoot:

- Determine reason for visit:
  - Concern about foot appearance/shoe wear
  - Pain related to foot deformity
  - Parental concern that flatfeet are abnormal and harmful if not treated[5]
- Assess developmental and past medical history: weakness, contractures, and/or spasticity may suggest neuromuscular cause
- Inquire about family history:
  - Familial hyperlaxity could suggest syndromes like Ehlers-Danlos or Marfan syndrome[6]
  - Some studies suggest flexible flatfeet may have a familial link[6,7]
- Assess for pain: location, duration, timing of symptoms
  - Location: Flexible flatfeet are typically painful or sore under the plantarmedial aspect of the midfoot and occasionally at the sinus tarsi. Patients with more rigid flatfeet typically present with pain in other locations as well.[8]
  - Duration/timing: Flatfoot pain is usually related to activity and relieved by rest. This is typically seen in both flexible and rigid flatfeet.[9] Night pain and pain at rest are not typical of flatfeet and warrant further investigation.
- Inquire regarding trauma: frequent ankle sprains may suggest tarsal coalition[10]

## Physical Examination

Assessment of pediatric flatfoot should include the following during the physical examination:

- Assess the child's lower extremity rotation and alignment from the hips to the ankles: genu valgus and external tibial torsion can make a flatfoot appear much more pronounced when standing.
- Inspection of the foot should occur in both a seated and a weight-bearing position.
  - Infants can have a flat arch in all positions.
  - Children often will have an arch while seated that flattens with standing.[8]
- Assess for Achilles tightness/contracture: the Silfverskiold test assesses ankle dorsiflexion with the knee in both flexion and extension to determine the source of contracture.
  - To clinically assess an Achilles contracture, the subtalar joint must be inverted to neutral and held in this position throughout examination.
  - If <10° of ankle dorsiflexion is obtained with the knee in both flexion and extension, the entire Achilles tendon is likely contracted.[8]
  - If >10° of ankle dorsiflexion is possible with the knee in flexion, yet dorsiflexion beyond 10° is not possible with the knee in extension, the gastrocnemius is likely affected.[8]
- Determine flexibility
  - Heel rise (**Fig. 1**)
    - Assess the hindfoot by examining the standing child from behind
    - While standing, the heel is typically in a valgus position (see **Fig. 1**A)
    - When the patient actively rises onto their toes for a heel rise, the medial longitudinal arch will elevate and the hindfoot will change from valgus to a neutral or varus position in flexible flatfoot deformities (see **Fig. 1**B)
    - If the foot is rigid, the arch will not elevate. In addition, the hindfoot will not correct and will remain in valgus during heel rise
- Gait
  - Assess for any unsteadiness, instability, asymmetry, or ataxia in gait that might suggest an underlying neurologic issue

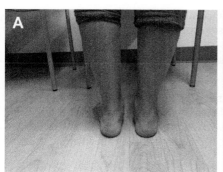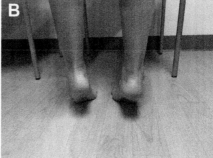

**Fig. 1.** Heel rise test to assess flexibility. While standing, there is minimal arch and the heel rests in valgus (*A*). When the patient actively rises up onto their toes for a heel rise, the medial longitudinal arch will elevate and the hindfoot will change from the valgus to a neutral or varus deformity in flexible flatfoot deformities (*B*).

o Observe the foot progression angle (angle of the foot relative to the line of progression), because patients with flatfeet typically have an outward foot progression angle

o Children should be asked to walk "normally" on their toes and their heels. This can help assess motor strength and rule out neurologic issues

• Determine location of pain and areas of tenderness

o Flexible flatfoot: pain usually localizes to the plantarmedial aspect of the foot but rarely tender on examination

o Tarsal coalition

■ Pain may localize to the anterolateral aspect of the foot just distal and anterior to the distal fibula in the setting of a calcaneonavicular coalition.

■ Pain may localize to a prominence just distal to the medial malleolus in the setting of a talocalcaneal coalition. This location is known as the "double medial malleolus."[11]

### Imaging

There is typically no need for imaging in the setting of an asymptomatic flexible flatfoot. In the symptomatic flexible flatfoot or the rigid flatfoot, imaging is typically obtained and modified based on the differential diagnosis.

| Images for typical pediatric flatfoot | Anteroposterior (AP)/lateral of the foot weight bearing AP of the ankle (to evaluate for ankle valgus) |
| --- | --- |
| If concern for calcaneonavicular coalition | External rotation 45° oblique view |
| If concern for talocalcaneal coalition | Harris view |
| If concern for accessory navicular | Internal rotation 45° oblique view |
| If concern for congenital vertical talus | Lateral of the foot in maximum plantarflexion (**Fig. 2**) |

The standing AP and lateral views can be used to assess several things, including calcaneal pitch, talocalcaneal angle, talonavicular coverage, and both anterior and lateral talus-first metatarsal (Meary) angles. The standing lateral view can also allow for visualization of a potential "anteater" sign, talar beaking, or C-sign in situations of tarsal coalition (**Fig. 3**).

Advanced imaging, such as computed tomography or MRI, is rarely indicated. However, these images can better evaluate tarsal coalition size and location and rule out coalitions in other locations of the foot.

## PHARMACOLOGIC TREATMENT OPTIONS

There are no known medication treatments that alter the natural history of pediatric flatfoot. Over-the-counter nonsteroidal anti-inflammatory medications (eg, ibuprofen, naproxen) may be used to manage activity-related pain associated with painful flatfeet. Narcotic pain medications are not recommended in any capacity for managing this condition.

## NONPHARMACOLOGIC TREATMENT OPTIONS

Most treatment algorithms for flexible flatfeet begin with simple observation. In the case of asymptomatic flexible flatfeet, parental education and reassurance are often

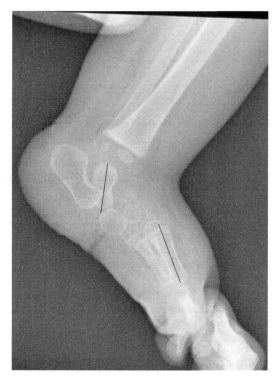

**Fig. 2.** Maximum plantarflexion lateral to evaluation for congenital vertical talus. In congenital vertical talus, there is persistent dorsal dislocation of the talonavicular joint on the max plantarflexion lateral. The lateral talus-first metatarsal angle is often increased and does not reduce to normal in the setting of a vertical talus.

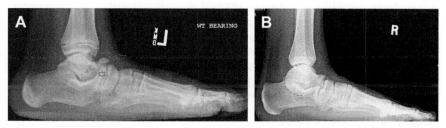

**Fig. 3.** Lateral standing radiograph of tarsal coalition. (A) The lateral view of a calcaneonavicular coalition demonstrates beaking of the talus (arrow) and the "anteater" sign or elongation of the anterior process of the calcaneus (star). (B) Lateral view of a foot with a talocalcaneal coalition demonstrating a C-sign.

all that is required for management (**Table 1**). Despite education that flatfeet may resolve with maturation and that there is no evidence that flatfoot deformity leads to a painful condition in adulthood, both parents and patients often seek treatment via orthotic arch supports.[12] A study published by Whitford and Esterman[13] in 2007 randomized 178 children aged 7 to 11 years to 2 different types of in-shoe orthoses, comparing them to a control group. No differences were found in the number of participants with foot pain between the 3 groups at either 3 or 12 months of follow-up.

| Table 1 | |
|---|---|
| Conservative treatment recommendations for flatfeet in children/adolescents | |
| **Type of Flatfoot in Children/Adolescent** | **Treatment** |
| Asymptomatic flexible flatfoot | Reassurance; no data to support orthoses |
| Symptomatic flexible flatfoot | Orthosis, but data are limited to support |
| Rigid flatfoot | Immobilization of tarsal coalition can help symptoms |

Thus, in-shoe arch-supporting orthoses are not routinely recommended to asymptomatic patients. There is no evidence that orthoses either correct deformity or prevent future symptoms.[12]

For symptomatic patients, some investigators advocate for the use of in-shoe prefabricated arch supports or custom orthoses in order to offload the plantarmedial soft tissues, invert the subtalar joint, and dorsiflex the talus.[3,8,13,14] The quality of evidence examining the effectiveness of arch supports and orthoses in symptomatic patients is poor. A *Cochrane Review* published in 2010 identified only 3 trials worthy of inclusion. Three hundred five patients were included in the review, which concluded that there is essentially no clear evidence to support the use of custom in-shoe orthoses in managing symptomatic flatfoot.[14] Despite the lack of clear evidence, arch-supporting orthoses are often recommended initially as low-cost conservative therapy for children with flexible flatfoot. Orthoses can be used in conjunction with heel cord stretching for patients with Achilles contractures often leading to symptom improvement.

Treatment of the rigid flatfoot depends on the underlying abnormality driving the hindfoot to stiffness. Corrective orthoses rely on flexibility of the flatfoot for correction, and are thus less useful in treating rigid flatfoot and often worsen symptoms. For tarsal coalitions, symptoms may improve with immobilization for 4 to 6 weeks, potentially staving off surgical management.[15]

Patients with spastic or flaccid flatfeet are managed based on their ambulatory status, symptoms, and presence/absence of intact protective sensation. Nonambulatory patients are typically not symptomatic from flatfeet and should be managed without orthoses, particularly if they lack protective sensation. Parents must be vigilant in monitoring for pressure sores when orthoses are implemented on a case-by-case basis. Ambulatory patients experiencing pain due to spastic flatfoot are difficult to actively brace against their spasticity: antispastic pharmacologic therapies and surgical intervention may offer more reliable outcomes.

## SURGICAL TREATMENT OPTIONS

Surgical management is not indicated for asymptomatic feet. For symptomatic feet, surgical management may be indicated when a reasonable trial of conservative management, typically for at least 6 months, has failed to improve the patient's symptoms.

Surgical procedures described for children with symptomatic flatfeet include the following:

- Osteotomies[3,4,16–18]
  - Calcaneal lengthening osteotomy (Evans procedure)
  - Calcaneal-cuboid-cuneiform osteotomy
  - Osteotomies in conjunction with soft tissue procedures
- Arthroereisis
- Arthrodesis

## Osteotomies

### Calcaneal (lateral column) lengthening osteotomy

Evans first described the calcaneal lengthening osteotomy in 1975 when he published preliminary qualitative results on 56 patients.[4] His theory was that varus and valgus were opposite deformities that developed as a result of relative length differences between the medial and lateral columns of the foot. He described elimination of excessive subtalar eversion and associated pain relief among his patients.

Mosca[3] further modified and developed the technique for the calcaneal lengthening procedure, publishing a subsequent series of 31 severe, symptomatic valgus flexible hindfeet managed with calcaneal lengthening osteotomy plus/minus medial cuneiform closing wedge plantarflexion osteotomy. As part of his correction, Mosca[3] released the lateral origin of the plantar fascia and abductor digiti minimi aponeurosis. He postulated that leaving the central and medial portions of the plantar fascia intact allowed for the windlass mechanism to propagate arch elevation and subtalar inversion.

### Modified Evans procedure pearls and pitfalls

- Protect peroneal tendons and sural nerve from injury on approach
- Divide the lateral plantar fascia and abductor digiti minimi aponeurosis (Mosca modification)
- Osteotomy planning
  - Clearly identify the middle and anterior facets, outlining the interval between them for the osteotomy to avoid iatrogenic injury to the subtalar joint surface
  - Orient the osteotomy with a slight oblique orientation from proximal-lateral to distal-medial in order to stay between the facets while advancing the osteotomy medially
- Fixation: There are multiple options for fixation of the osteotomy. The authors typically use a Kirschner wire because it can be removed leaving no retained implants in children/adolescents.
  - After completing the osteotomy but before placing the bone graft, place a retrograde Kirschner wire across the calcaneocuboid (CC) joint with an orientation on the AP radiograph that will allow it to be used to both hold the CC joint reduced and pin the bone graft in to position within the osteotomy site.
  - Once the graft is in place, the Kirschner wire can be advanced (**Fig. 4**A, B).
- Use a lamina spreader or Hintermann retractor to assess the graft size needed to reduce the talonavicular joint.
- Use a trapezoid-shaped bone graft in order to introduce both lengthening and adduction via an opening wedge. Mosca advises use of a tricortical iliac crest graft (allograft or autograft) measuring 10 to 12 mm in length laterally and 4 to 6 mm medially.[3]
- Soft tissue adjuncts as advocated by Mosca[3]
  - Isolated soft tissue procedures are rarely successful but are often needed in conjunction with bony procedures.[7]
  - Peroneal tendons: z-lengthen if they resist lateral osteotomy distraction, particularly in cerebral palsy patients with spastic peroneal tendons
  - Posterior tibial tendons: may advance to remove excess length
  - Talonavicular joint capsule: plantar-medial plication in order to remove redundancy
  - Achilles tendon: lengthening performed if passive ankle dorsiflexion is less than 10° with the knee extended following calcaneal lengthening

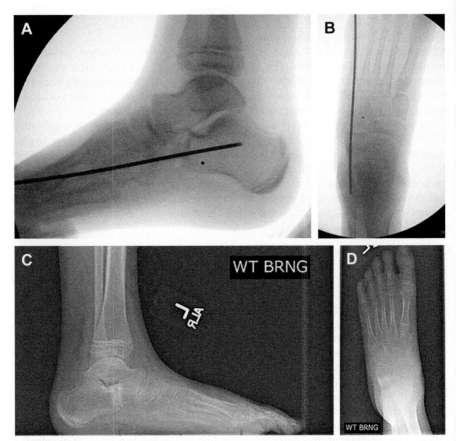

Fig. 4. Calcaneal lengthening osteotomy. A Kirschner wire can be used to hold the bone graft in place in children. It should be placed from the cuboid into the distal aspect of the calcaneus before opening the osteotomy site to avoid calcaneal cuboid subluxation (A, B). The wires can be removed in clinic at 4 postoperative weeks. Weight-bearing films can be adequately obtained around 8 weeks postoperatively (C, D).

- Residual forefoot supination: if rigid, should be corrected with a plantarmedial medial cuneiform closing wedge plantar-flexion osteotomy
- Postoperative immobilization
  - Cast for ~4 weeks; non-weight-bearing
  - Remove Kirschner wire around 4 weeks postoperatively. At this visit, the patient can be transitioned to a short leg walking cast for an additional 3 to 4 weeks. First weight-bearing radiographs are typically done around 8 weeks (see Fig. 4C, D).
  - In neuromuscular disorders, the patient can be transitioned into braces at the 4- or 8-week mark postoperatively depending on the weight-bearing ability of the child.

### Calcaneal-cuboid-cuneiform osteotomy

In 1998, Rathjen and Mubarak[17] reported the details of severe valgus deformity correction in 24 feet (16 children) using a combination of a medial displacement calcaneal osteotomy, an opening wedge cuboid osteotomy, and a closing wedge plantar medial cuneiform osteotomy.[17] The theory behind this combination of osteotomies is to avoid disrupting articular surfaces.[17] The medial displacement calcaneal osteotomy is intended to functionally correct calcaneal valgus, and a closing wedge of bone may be removed through the lateral calcaneal exposure. The cuboid opening wedge osteotomy drives the forefoot into adduction, and the plantarflexion medial cuneiform osteotomy both introduces increased arch height and pronates the forefoot. Associated procedures in this series included gastrocnemius recession (15), medial talonavicular capsular reefing (14), and peroneal lengthening (13) as soft tissue adjuncts to deformity correction.

### Calcaneal-cuboid-cuneiform osteotomy pearls and pitfalls

- Protect peroneal tendons and sural nerve from injury on approach laterally
- The calcaneal bone cut is made with an oscillating saw. The medial cortical wall of the osteotomy may be completed more safely using an osteotome from the lateral side.
- A small medial-based wedge is removed from the more proximal aspect of the calcaneus to aid in the calcaneal slide and deformity correction.
- The cuboid bone cut is made with an oscillating saw and completed dorsally with an osteotome.
- The plantar wedge removed from the medial cuneiform can be used as an autograft for the opening wedge on the cuboid.
- Kirschner wire fixation for this osteotomy is similar to that as described in the calcaneal lengthening osteotomy. The calcaneus can be fixed with Kirschner wires as well, placed into the heel and exiting toward the sinus tarsi.
- Postoperative casting is similar to that as described above.

## Soft Tissue Procedures

Of note, soft tissue adjunct procedures, including Achilles tendon lengthening, gastrocnemius recession, medial talonavicular capsular reefing, posterior tibialis tendon advancement, and peroneal lengthening, may be necessary in order to balance the foot when performing osteotomy-mediated correction. These procedures have not been studied in the pediatric population independent of their parent procedures. Please reference specific procedural pearls and pitfalls for more information.

## Arthroereisis

A less invasive procedure termed arthroereisis, intended to restrict subtalar joint motion without injuring the joint, normalizing dynamic anatomic relationships, has been popularized more recently. A bioabsorbable, silicone, or titanium cone-shaped implant, approximately 6 to 8 mm in diameter (manufacturer dependent), is surgically inserted within the "extra-articular" portion of the sinus tarsi, restricting pronation of the subtalar joint, elevating the arch, and improving talonavicular congruity. The indications for this type of procedure remain controversial.[14] The authors do not routinely use this type of treatment.

### Arthroereisis pearls and pitfalls

Recommendations of technique based on previously described literature.[19]

- A lateral incision is made over the sinus tarsi. Blunt dissection is used to avoid injury to cutaneous nerves.
- A blunt probe is placed into the sinus tarsi from lateral to medial just anterior to the posterior facet. Some investigators will place the probe percutaneously through the medial aspect of the foot just superior to the posterior tibial tendon.

- Various sizing guides can then be used with the hindfoot held in a near neutral alignment.
- Proper implant placement can be determined radiographically: On the AP image of the foot, the implant should be 1 cm medial to the lateral edge of the calcaneus, and the total implant should be less than half of the width of the talus. On the lateral image of the foot, the implant should be seated directly on the floor of the sinus tarsi.

### Arthrodesis

Triple arthrodesis, defined as arthrodesis of the subtalar, talonavicular, and CC joints, was introduced as a possible treatment option in the 1960s in response to failures of limited talonavicular arthrodesis. At this time, the biomechanics of the deformity were less well understood. Seitz and Carpenter[20] first published a long-term follow-up series in 1974, detailing a 10-year review (minimum 2-year follow-up) of triple arthrodesis performed at a single institution. At final follow-up, 90% of patients had no or negligible residual pain, although 57% had residual deformity. The patients included in this study, however, were poorly defined and heterogeneous in their indications for arthrodesis.

Triple arthrodesis is rarely used in the treatment of pediatric flatfoot. Although there is little published regarding treatment in pediatric patients, this surgical treatment has been discussed in the treatment of the rigid neurologic flatfoot.[21]

### Surgical Treatment of Rigid Flatfeet

A rigid flatfoot that results from a coincident valgus hindfoot and talocalcaneal coalition, although uncommon, may be approached with calcaneal lengthening osteotomy with or without simultaneous coalition excision depending on several characteristics in Mosca and Bevan.[22] These observations are based on a limited series detailing a series of 13 successfully treated patients with rigid flatfoot due to talocalcaneal coalition: only one patient required fusion for degenerative talonavicular changes present upon the child's presentation and only one patient was dissatisfied on intermediate-term follow-up.[22] In some patients with significant heel valgus (>16°), and a small middle facet coalition, treatment with coalition resection and calcaneal lengthening osteotomy can be successful.

**Table 2**
**Reported complications of surgical procedures**

| Surgical Procedure | Reported Complications |
|---|---|
| Calcaneal lengthening osteotomy[3,8,12,18] | Persistent pain<br>Undercorrection<br>Overcorrection<br>Graft slippage/collapse<br>CC subluxation |
| Triple C osteotomy[17,18] | Persistent pain<br>Undercorrection<br>Graft slippage/collapse |
| Arthroereisis[28,29] | Implant extrusion leading to unplanned removal<br>Undercorrection<br>Implant resorption<br>Inflammatory reactions<br>Persistent pain |
| Arthrodesis[30] | Adjacent joint degenerative changes<br>Residual deformity<br>Persistent pain |

Further discussion of surgical treatment techniques for rigid flatfoot management is beyond the scope of this article. However, techniques of coalition resection[23,24] and congenital vertical talus[25-27] treatment have been well described.

## TREATMENT COMPLICATIONS

Treatment complications are outlined in **Table 2**. In addition to these complications related to specific flatfoot reconstruction procedures, it is of utmost importance to

**Table 3**
**Outcomes reported by procedure for symptomatic flatfoot**

| Surgical Procedure | Reported Outcomes |
|---|---|
| Calcaneal lengthening osteotomy | • Phillips[16] published a long-term (13 y) follow-up series reporting "very good" or "good" results in 17/23 feet; only 3/23 were noted to have persistence or recurrence of pain associated with recurrent hindfoot valgus<br>• Mosca[3] reported successful results in 29/31 feet. Importantly, most of the patients included in Mosca's series had neuromuscular flatfoot, an indication that Evans warned to approach with caution given his marginal results among patients with spastic disorders and myelomeningocele |
| Triple C osteotomy | • Rathjen and Mubarak[17] report outcomes graded as "excellent" or "good" in all but one case (23/24) with an average of 18-mo follow-up[17]; 79% of patients' lateral talo-first metatarsal angles were corrected to within normal limits on final weight-bearing radiographs |
| Arthroereisis[28,29] | • Sustainable clinical improvement of standing heel valgus angle and radiographic improvement of lateral talo-first metatarsal angle have been reported following arthroereisis for flexible flatfeet with 4-y follow-up[29]<br>• A subsequent critical literature review of available case series and re-ports (76 total small studies identified) presented satisfactory out-comes in 79%–100% of patients despite a complication rate of 5%–19% among patients undergoing arthroereisis.[28] Radiographic data reported in the arthroereisis literature[20] indicate an increase in static arch height and improved subtalar joint congruity |
| Arthrodesis[30] | • In a cohort of 57 patients, Saltzman and colleagues[30] published 25- and 44-y average follow-up data following triple arthrodesis, usually indicated for neuromuscular foot imbalance<br>  ○ At 25 y, 45% of patients had persistent/recurrent foot pain, and 32% required walking support devices<br>  ○ Outcomes at 44 y continued to deteriorate. In all patients, degen-erative changes were radiographically apparent within the tibiotalar joint at 44-y follow-up. Similar progressive arthritic changes were found in the naviculocuneiform and tarsometatarsal joints<br>  ○ Despite persistent and slowly progressive disability, 95% of patients were satisfied with their long-term outcomes, likely owing to the most commonly included indication for intervention, the neuromuscular foot imbalance due to poliomyelitis<br>• This long-term evidence of adjacent joint arthritis, even in a low-demand population, following triple arthrodesis is a cause for concern in pediatric flatfoot. If realignment of the symptomatic, flexible hindfoot is possible without sacrificing hindfoot joints in an ambulatory patient, adjacent joint degeneration can be avoided. Thus, arthrodesis is currently used as a salvage procedure for most patients or primarily used in neurologic flatfoot |

correctly identify the less common rigid flatfoot, because treatment approach will be different.

## EVALUATION OF OUTCOMES
### Outcome by Procedure

Very few long-term outcomes exist regarding surgical treatment of the pediatric flat-foot. **Table 3** is a summary of surgical outcomes reported by procedure.

### Outcome Comparison Between Calcaneal Lengthening and Calcaneo-Cuboid-Cuneiform Osteotomy

One study attempts to address the question of which osteotomy combination provides the most consistent correction: a retrospective comparative series (Level III evidence) detailed by Moraleda and colleagues[18] in 2012. Clinical and radiographic outcomes were compared in 63 total children's feet: 30 underwent flatfoot correction with calcaneo-cuboid-cuneiform osteotomies and 33 underwent calcaneal lengthening osteotomy. No differences were observed in clinical outcomes scores. Both the AP talo-first metatarsal angle and degree of talonavicular coverage were found to have been better corrected with calcaneal lengthening osteotomy. The calcaneo-cuboid-cuneiform osteotomy combination, however, does not generate subluxation at the CC joint that the calcaneal lengthening osteotomy does; subluxation was found to occur at a 52% rate among patients treated with a calcaneal lengthening osteotomy.

Both procedures facilitate adequate deformity correction and symptom relief in the appropriately selected symptomatic patient. It is unclear what long-term impact, if any, CC subluxation may cause in patients treated with calcaneal lengthening. Importantly, "mild" radiographic changes are briefly noted among an unspecified number of patients with "good" results in the 13-year average follow-up series reported by Phillips.[16]

## SUMMARY

Pediatric flatfeet are common. In young patients, it is often physiologic, and natural history studies suggest improvement over time in most children.[1] It is critical to differentiate flexible from rigid flatfeet and to assess for associated Achilles contracture with a careful history, physical examination, and initial radiographs. Asymptomatic flatfeet do not require any treatment. Although there are limited data, nonsurgical management of the symptomatic flatfeet, both flexible and rigid, should be exhausted before considering surgical intervention. Surgical management with joint-preserving, deformity-corrective techniques is typically used for pediatric flexible flatfeet in conjunction with deformity-specific soft tissue procedures. True long-term outcome studies following surgical treatment are lacking in the pediatric population.

## REFERENCES

1. Pfeiffer M, Kotz R, Ledl T, et al. Prevalence of flat foot in preschool-aged children. Pediatrics 2006;118(2):634–9.
2. Villarroya MA, Esquivel JM, Tomás C, et al. Assessment of the medial longitudinal arch in children and adolescents with obesity: footprints and radiographic study. Eur J Pediatr 2008;168(5):559–67.
3. Mosca VS. Calcaneal lengthening for valgus deformity of the hindfoot. Results in children who had severe, symptomatic flatfoot and skewfoot. J Bone Joint Surg 1995;77(4):500–12.

4. Evans D. Calcaneo-valgus deformity. J Bone Joint Surg Br 1975;57(3):270–8.
5. Kim HW, Weinstein SL. Flatfoot in children: differential diagnosis and management. Curr Orthop 2000;14:441–7.
6. Harris EJ, Vanore JV, Thomas JL, et al. Diagnosis and treatment of pediatric flatfoot. J Foot Ankle Surg 2004;43(6):341–73.
7. Mosca VS. Flexible flatfoot in children and adolescents. J Child Orthop 2010;4(2): 107–21.
8. Bouchard M, Mosca VS. Flatfoot deformity in children and adolescents: surgical indications and management. J Am Acad Orthop Surg 2014;22(10):623–32.
9. Sheikh Taha AM, Feldman DS. Painful flexible flatfoot. Foot Ankle Clin 2015;20(4): 693–704.
10. Snyder RB, Lipscomb AB. The relationship of tarsal coalitions to ankle sprains in athletes. Am J Sports Med 1981;9(5):313–7.
11. Rocchi V, Huang M-T, Bomar JD, et al. The "Double Medial Malleolus": a new physical finding in talocalcaneal coalition. J Pediatr Orthop 2016;1.
12. Kwon JY, Myerson MS. Management of the flexible flat foot in the child: a focus on the use of osteotomies for correction. Foot Ankle Clin 2010;15(2):309–22.
13. Whitford D, Esterman A. A randomized controlled trial of two types of in-shoe orthoses in children with flexible excess pronation of the feet. Foot Ankle Int 2007; 28(6):715–23.
14. Rome K, Ashford RL, Evans A. Non-surgical interventions for paediatric pes planus. Cochrane Database Syst Rev 2010;(7):CD006311.
15. Bohne WH. Tarsal coalition. Curr Opin Pediatr 2001;13(1):29–35.
16. Phillips GE. A review of elongation of os calcis for flat feet. J Bone Joint Surg Br 1983;65(1):15–8.
17. Rathjen KE, Mubarak SJ. Calcaneal-cuboid-cuneiform osteotomy for the correction of valgus foot deformities in children. J Pediatr Orthop 1998;18(6):775–82.
18. Moraleda L, Salcedo M, Bastrom TP, et al. Comparison of the calcaneo-cuboid-cuneiform osteotomies and the calcaneal lengthening osteotomy in the surgical treatment of symptomatic flexible flatfoot. J Pediatr Orthop 2012;32(8):821–9.
19. Scharer BM, Black BE, Sockrider N. Treatment of painful pediatric flatfoot with Maxwell-Brancheau subtalar arthroereisis implant a retrospective radiographic review. Foot Ankle Spec 2010;3(2):67–72.
20. Seitz DG, Carpenter EB. Triple arthrodesis in children: a ten-year review. South Med J 1974;67(12):1420–4.
21. Dare DM, Dodwell ER. Pediatric flatfoot: cause, epidemiology, assessment, and treatment. Curr Opin Pediatr 2014;26(1):93–100.
22. Mosca VS, Bevan WP. Talocalcaneal tarsal coalitions and the calcaneal lengthening osteotomy: the role of deformity correction. J Bone Joint Surg Am 2012; 94(17):1584–94.
23. Mubarak SJ, Patel PN, Upasani VV, et al. Calcaneonavicular coalition: treatment by excision and fat graft. J Pediatr Orthop 2009;29(5):418–26.
24. Gantsoudes GD, Roocroft JH, Mubarak SJ. Treatment of talocalcaneal coalitions. J Pediatr Orthop 2012;32(3):301–7.
25. Dobbs MB, Purcell DB, Nunley R, et al. Early results of a new method of treatment for idiopathic congenital vertical talus. J Bone Joint Surg 2006;88(6):1192–200.
26. Dobbs MB, Purcell DB, Nunley R, et al. Early results of a new method of treatment for idiopathic congenital vertical talus. Surgical technique. J Bone Joint Surg 2007;89(Suppl 2 Pt.1):111–21.

27. Yang JS, Dobbs MB. Treatment of congenital vertical talus: comparison of minimally invasive and extensive soft-tissue release procedures at minimum five-year follow-up. J Bone Joint Surg Am 2015;97(16):1354–65.
28. Metcalfe SA, Bowling FL, Reeves ND. Subtalar joint arthroereisis in the management of pediatric flexible flatfoot: a critical review of the literature. Foot Ankle Int 2011;32(12):1127–39.
29. Giannini BS, Ceccarelli F, Benedetti MG, et al. Surgical treatment of flexible flatfoot in children a four-year follow-up study. J Bone Joint Surg 2001;83A(Suppl 2 Pt 2):73–9.
30. Saltzman CL, Fehrle MJ, Cooper RR, et al. Triple arthrodesis: twenty-five and forty-four-year average follow-up of the same patients. J Bone Joint Surg Am 1999;81(10):1391–402.

Printed and bound by CPI Group (UK) Ltd, Croydon, CR0 4YY

08/05/2025

01864702-0001